A Profile in Alternative Medicine

A Profile in Alternative Medicine

The Eclectic Medical College of Cincinnati, 1845–1942

JOHN S. HALLER, JR.

THE KENT STATE UNIVERSITY PRESS

Kent, Ohio, and London, England

© 1999 by The Kent State University Press, Kent, Ohio 44242
All rights reserved
Library of Congress Catalog Card Number 98-43302
ISBN 0-87338-610-8
Manufactured in the United States of America

04 03 02 01 00 99   5 4 3 2 1

Library of Congress Cataloging-in-Publication Data

Haller, John S.
    A profile in alternative medicine : the Eclectic Medical College
of Cincinnati, 1845–1942 / John S. Haller, Jr.
        p.   cm.
    Includes bibliographical references and index.
    ISBN 0-87338-610-8 (cloth : alk. paper) ∞
    1. Eclectic Medical College—History.   2. Medicine, Eclectic—
History.   3. Medical colleges—Ohio—Cincinnati—History 19th
century.   4. Medical colleges—Ohio—Cincinnati—History 20th
century.   I. Title.   II. Title: Eclectic Medical College of
Cincinnati, 1845–1942.
    [DNLM: 1. Eclectic Medical College.   2. Alternative Medicine—
education—Ohio.   3. Schools, Medical—history—Ohio.
4. Eclecticism—history—Ohio.   WB 18 H185p   1999]
RV101.C5H35   1999
610'.71'177178—dc21
DNLM/DLC
for Library of Congress   98-43302
                                                                CIP

British Library Cataloging-in-Publication data are available.

For

George Callcott

If you wish to ascertain the truths of the Christian religion, you do not ask the infidel. . . . For like reasons, if you care to understand the principles of the Eclectic school of medicine, quiz not the old school doctor, for he is both inimical to and ignorant of them. . . . With but few exceptions, when they do study the "specific" or Eclectic practice of medicine, they do so from the standpoint of partisan prejudice, as an atheist studies the Bible.

—Albert H. Collins

Eclectic Medical College Bulletin, 1914

Contents

Illustrations

Acknowledgments

THOSE TO WHOM I am indebted include colleagues John Jackson, Kyle Perkins, Benjamin A. Shepherd, John Yopp, David P. Werlich, John Y. Simon, David L. Wilson, James Smith Allen, Kay J. Carr, Howard W. Allen, Donald S. Detweiler, John E. Dotson, H. Arnold Barton, H. Browning Carrott, Julius E. Thompson, Margorie Morgan, Robbie Lieberman, Rachel Stocking, Edward O'Day, Michael C. Batinski, Tien-Wei Wu, Theodore Weeks, Phillip V. Davis, Mary Ellen McElligott, Barbara Mason, and William and Jo Holohan. Special thanks go to Alex Berman who, over many years, has been the standard-bearer of scholarship in the history of botanical medicine and who, more recently, has become a good friend and colleague. I have treasured his scholarship as I now treasure his advice and friendship. I am also grateful to my wife, Robin, who has offered inspiration, encouragement, criticism, and substantial assistance, including editing numerous drafts and indexing the finished manuscript.

Like most authors of historical works, I am especially obligated to the historian-collector-librarians and their professional staffs. Their generosity of time and experienced assistance has made it possible for me to enrich my understanding of the subject matter and to carry out the necessary research. In this regard, I extend my sincere gratitude to librarian and director Michael A. Flannery and staff members Mary Lee Schmidt, Betsy Kruthoffer, Rose Marie Weckenmann, Anna Lee Schmidt, and Victor R. Perry of the Lloyd Library and Museum in Cincinnati, Ohio. Each provided invaluable assistance in opening to me the resources of the Lloyd Library and its wonderful collection on the botanic reformers in American medicine. Without their help this book could not have been written. Michael Flannery deserves special thanks. He provided me with the full support of the Lloyd staff and his own personal assistance. His ongoing research on John Uri Lloyd and his knowledge of the Lloyd family helped measurably in the completion of this project. I also wish to thank Dr. Sam Rockwern, M.D., who graduated from the University of Cincinnati Medical School and who taught at EMC in its last semester in 1939. I drew upon his memory of specific individuals and events to validate my own historical observations and conclusions.

Other librarians to whom I am indebted include Kathy Fahey, Mary R. Taylor, Karen Drickamer, James W. Fox, Mary Anne Fox, Kimbra Stout, Andrew Tax, Harry Davis, Iva McRoberts, and Carolyn Synder from the Morris Library of Southern Illinois University, Carbondale; Connie Poole and Jeff Martin from the Southern Illinois University School of Medicine Library; Roger Guard from the University of Cincinnati Medical Library; and Peter Hirtle and Margaret Kaiser at the National Library of Medicine. Finally, my gratitude would not be complete without mentioning the fine libraries whose collections I used. These include the Medical Library of Southern Illinois University School of Medicine, Springfield; the University of Illinois Library, Champaign-Urbana; the University of Oregon Medical School Library, Eugene; Kent State University Library; Indiana State University Library, Terre Haute; Indiana State Library, Indianapolis; the University of California at Irvine Medical Sciences Library; Indiana University Library, Bloomington; Johns Hopkins University Library, Baltimore; the Library of Congress; the National Library of Medicine, Bethesda, Maryland; and the Center for Research Libraries, Chicago.

Finally, my acknowledgments would not be complete without expressing my debt to George Callcott, emeritus professor of history at the University of Maryland, to whom I credit my passion for historical research and writing. Before leaving Maryland for my first teaching position, he met me one last time in his office, and, wishing me well, challenged me by saying that I was "worth at least seven books." Although he doesn't remember ever having said it, I do, and his challenge has served me well through the years. This book is dedicated to my mentor and friend, George Callcott.

Introduction

THE ECLECTIC MEDICAL INSTITUTE, known by its friends as "Old EMI" (and "Old EMC" when reorganized in 1910), was an American institution in origin, concept, and practice, portrayed throughout its ninety-four-year history as a bastion of freedom in medical thought and teaching. Its early success, adversity, and ultimate failure is the story of a struggle by a few determined reformers to build a school based on plant medicines, maintenance of the body's vital force, avoidance of depletive remedies, and the dual concepts of specific diagnosis and specific medication. Fond of their origins, the faculty embodied in their teachings and writings a protest against the hegemony of allopathic medicine. Reminiscent of Luther's ninety-five theses against indulgences were their protests against the indiscriminate use of minerals and the reckless employment of bleeding, cupping, and blistering, practices they perceived as dominating orthodox therapeutics in the late eighteenth and early nineteenth centuries. Teaching a milder method of drug therapy and a more intelligent use of the materia medica, they claimed to have forced allopathy to reform itself while, at the same time, establishing for themselves an independent school of therapeutics.

The interested reader should find several significant aspects to this study. First, it recounts the history of eclectic medicine that, along with Thomsonism, homeopathy, hydropathy, and physio-medicalism, represented the earliest wave of medical sectarianism in the nineteenth century. In its peak years, ten thousand or more eclectic physicians practiced in the United States. Second, although historians have explained the philosophies behind these unorthodox medical *systems*, there exist no complete histories of individual institutions that adhered to these beliefs. Unlike most sectarian schools that closed without leaving many documents, EMC left student records, faculty files, deans' papers, minutes of the board of trustees meetings and of its executive committee, and the minutes of the school's alumni association. These materials, archived at the Lloyd Library and Museum in Cincinnati, provide an important window into sectarian medicine's many challenges; the character of the school's students, faculty, and alumni; and its unsuccessful struggle to obtain a class-A rating by the American Medical Association's Council on Medical Education. The history of the school is doubly important since EMC served as the mecca of eclectic thinking in the nineteenth and twentieth centuries, held in high esteem as the "mother institute" of reformed medicine.[1]

Finally, the college attracted three distinctly different student populations: true believers in medical eclecticism who, upon graduation, became respected family practitioners; high-risk students who, unable to succeed at medical schools elsewhere, viewed EMC as a school of last chance; and well-educated sons of Jewish immigrants who, because of either exclusion or quota restrictions at other medical colleges, chose the college as a back door into medicine. Although its early years witnessed significant numbers of students dedicated to practicing reform medicine, motives other than eclecticism influenced later ranks of matriculants. By 1920, not more than half of EMC's graduating classes were true believers in eclectic medical philosophy.

The history of the Eclectic Medical College represents the continuation of a story first discussed in my *Medical Protestants: The Eclectics in American Medicine, 1825–1939* (1994), which focused principally upon the philosophy of eclecticism but addressed EMC as the representative institution for much of eclectic thinking. By treating the college in greater detail in this present work, I have built on the only other institutional history of the college, Harvey Wickes Felter's *History of the Eclectic Medical Institute* (1902). I have not attempted to rewrite the school's earlier history beyond what Felter and I have already recounted. Instead, I have chosen to focus principally on the years after 1890 as the college attempted to accommodate to the rigors of academic medicine.

One last point is worth mentioning. In the latter part of the nineteenth century, chiropractic and osteopathic medicine emerged as alternative therapeutic systems. The impact of these two groups, while significant, weighed more heavily in the late twentieth century than in the years covered by this study. For that reason, I have chosen to exclude them.

CHAPTER ONE

Cincinnati's Medical Establishment

T HE CITY OF CINCINNATI, situated halfway between Pittsburgh at the head of the Ohio River and Cairo at its junction with the Mississippi, is part of the Miami country explored in 1751 by Christopher Gist, an agent for the Ohio Company. The original settlement, surrounded by a well-defined circle of hills, commenced in December 1788 with a population of eleven families and twenty-four unmarried men. A year later, the newly formed United States built Fort Washington on a site that is today Third Street. Threatened by Indians and disease during its early years, the settlement grew quickly as peace and security came to the region. By 1795, the town contained ninety-four cabins, ten frame houses, and five hundred inhabitants. With the boundaries of Ohio determined in 1802, two significant events occurred the following year: the town of Cincinnati was incorporated by the territorial legislature, and state government began operation. By 1805, the population had increased to 960 inhabitants and, in 1819, the state legislature granted a charter incorporating Cincinnati as a city.[1]

The nickname "Queen City" appears to have been given to Cincinnati before 1834, but the actual origin will probably never be known. In all likelihood, it derived from the city's strategic river location for moving merchandise and raw materials along the nation's principal water routes. Early in the city's history, large grocery houses, wholesale dry-goods stores, and pork-packing plants lined Front, Broadway, and Main Streets, which crowded close to the public landing. The city's waterfront teemed with boats and passengers while roustabouts moved cotton, barrels, and other goods across gangplanks. Beyond the landing, flatboats, barges, and other craft transported

people and cargo up and down the river. Steamboats appeared in growing numbers in the 1820s, and by midcentury the city had become a
center of commerce and industry for the West. After the Civil War,
steamboats continued to draw travelers for overnight passenger service, but railroads soon took over the movement of tonnage.[2]

The early settlers of the city came principally from the middle
and northern Atlantic states and secondarily from the South. In later
years, they came more directly from Europe, especially Germany, Ire-
land, England, Scotland, and Wales. From 1825 onward, German mi-
gration outstripped all others, with the Irish close behind. Cincinnati
became a city of editors, publicists, musicians, scientists, divines, and
pork packers. The black population, chiefly emancipated slaves and
their offspring, arrived in small but steady numbers from Kentucky
and Virginia. Census information reported a population of 24,831 in
1830; 46,338 in 1840; and 115,438 in 1850, including 3,172 blacks.[3]
Occupations and trades in 1850 included 176 attorneys; 227 barbers;
713 blacksmiths; 1,569 boot and shoe makers; 672 butchers; 327 coffee
house keepers; 126 brewers; 533 grocers; 28 policemen; 278 doctors; and 153 druggists.[4] By then, too, the city touted 91 churches and
3 synagogues; 19 public schools; 3 liberal arts colleges; 4 mercantile
colleges; 5 theological schools; 1 law school; and 4 medical colleges.[5]

EARLY DOCTORS

The earliest medical care for the pioneers of the Queen City came
by way of surgeons attached to the regular army of the United States
who opened their army hospital chests to sick civilians and who, upon
leaving the military, established practices in and around the village.
The earliest military surgeons included Richard Allison, John Car-
michael, Joseph Phillips, John Elliot, and John Sellman. These were
replaced by citizen-physicians, the first of whom was William Burnet
in 1789, followed in quick succession by Calvin Morrell, John Hole,
John Cramer, John Stites, Jr., John Blackburn, Samuel Ramsey, William Goforth, and his friend and pupil Daniel Drake.[6]

Daniel Drake (1785–1852), who received the first medical diploma
awarded west of the Allegheny Mountains, began practicing medicine
in May 1804 at the age of nineteen, as partner to his former preceptor. A year later, he traveled to Philadelphia to study medicine more

formally at the University of Pennsylvania. In 1807, he returned to Cincinnati to take over Goforth's practice but went back briefly to Philadelphia in the fall of 1815 to complete the doctor of medicine degree. Over the next several decades, he had a role in the creation of several medical departments, hospitals, and affiliated units, including Transylvania University in Lexington, Kentucky, the first medical school west of the Alleghenies; the Medical College of Ohio, the second medical school of the West, which in 1896 became the Medical Department of the University of Cincinnati; the old Commercial Hospital and Lunatic Asylum, the predecessor to the University of Cincinnati Hospital; the Eye Infirmary of Cincinnati; the Western Museum Society (for which he hired John James Audubon); and the medical department of Cincinnati College, which he founded in 1835 after being expelled from the Medical College of Ohio. He authored *Notices Concerning Cincinnati* (1810), which provided an account of the town and of plants indigenous to the region; *Natural and Statistical View, or Pictures of Cincinnati and the Miami County* (1815), which he used to encourage settlement; the *Western Journal of the Medical and Physical Sciences* (1827–38), which he published and edited; *Practical Essays on Medical Education, and the Medical Profession, in the United States* (1832); and his most important work, *A Systematic Treatise, Historical, Etiological and Practical on the Principal Diseases of the Interior Valley of North America* (1850), which he wrote while teaching at the Louisville Medical Institute.[7]

According to Drake, every one of the city's physicians was also a country practitioner who rode twelve to fifteen miles on bridle paths to visit sick patients. The typical charge was twenty-five cents a mile, "one half being deducted and the other paid in provender for his horse or produce for his family." Doctors bled and cupped their patients, practiced dentistry, acted as their own apothecaries, and charged patients additional amounts for any personal services performed. For example, they charged twenty-five cents for a bleeding; the same amount for a draught of paregoric and antimonial wine; fifty cents for a vermifuge or blister; seventy-five cents for an ounce of Peruvian bark; and a dollar for sitting up all night with a patient. Although physicians carried medicines with them on their visits, they were just as apt to return home from a visit, compound a special mixture, and send it along to the patient.[8]

MEDICAL DEMOCRACY

Medical education in eighteenth-century America was a relatively simple affair. A student desiring a career in medicine apprenticed himself to a willing physician who served as preceptor and instructed him in the accumulated wisdom and experience of the practice. For a period of four to seven years, the apprentice remained a part of the doctor's household; kept case books; read from available medical texts; learned how to prepare drugs; followed the doctor on his visits; helped to bleed, blister, and pull teeth; and generally learned the art and science of medicine. As one might imagine, the quality of apprenticeship varied with the educational background of the student, the nature of the preceptor's practice, the availability of relevant medical texts, and the quality of supervision. American society needed doctors before there was an adequate way of educating them, and apprenticeship afforded a workable solution.[9]

Besides these home-grown physicians, some supplemented their apprenticeship with education abroad—at the University of Leyden in Holland, Hôtel Dieu of Paris, Guy's or St. Thomas's Hospital in London, Dublin's Meath Hospital, or the Edinburgh Royal Infirmary. There they took private courses (such as William Hunter's theater in Covent Garden), enrolled for a medical degree, walked the hospital wards witnessing operations and dissections, and, in general, observed and studied a greater variety of diseases than were seen in a preceptor's private practice. Upon returning to America, many of these same young men, inspired by what they saw and did abroad, organized medical schools patterned on European models. By 1800, ten medical departments, in conjunction with hospitals and established universities, provided the eastern seaboard states with a high level of clinical and didactic instruction.[10]

The system of apprenticeship adapted comfortably to the establishment of medical departments. The term of apprenticeship shortened to three years, with the understanding that the aspiring young doctor would divide his time between a preceptor and a didactic education. The faculty of these early schools gave lectures in anatomy, chemistry, theory and practice of medicine, surgery, medical jurisprudence, materia medica and botany, midwifery, and diseases of women and children. To overcome the lack of textbooks, medical training included two terms of the same subject matter, the rationale being that students who found it difficult to cover the prescribed material in the first term had the opportunity to complete their studies in the second.[11]

Along with the salutary quality of university affiliation, the faculty in these medical departments enjoyed a high degree of autonomy; in terms of financial responsibility and supervision they had only nominal contact with the academic institution. Having received authority from a university to grant degrees, doctors operated a virtual *imperium in imperio,* setting their own salaries, tuition, and curriculum. The income for the faculty derived mainly from lecture tickets, although occasionally state legislatures permitted the use of lotteries to raise funds. Because of their heavy dependence on lecture fees, faculty were sometimes tempted to admit candidates on the basis of their ability to pay rather than on their potential as doctors.

The founding of the proprietary College of Medicine of Maryland in 1807 led to a new indigenous model of American medical education that spawned dozens of imitators in the states and territories west of the Appalachians. Unlike the Maryland college, which was actually well managed, many imitators lacked equipment, books, and qualified teachers, and only a few could boast even a nominal hospital affiliation. Except for occasional dissections, which some schools treated as optional, the curriculum was wholly didactic. Organized on a for-profit basis, these colleges operated as stock companies and paid an annual dividend to shareholders. Faculty brought and sold their teaching chairs, which were sources of both status and income, and relied on former students to send consultations their way out of school loyalty. By 1877, fewer than twenty of the sixty-five medical colleges in existence were connected with institutions of higher learning.[12]

As these proprietary schools proliferated and competition increased, faculties chose to capture their share of the student market through a combination of minimal entrance requirements, shortened curricula and terms, reduced matriculation and lecture fees, and lowered graduation expectations. In the absence of clinical facilities and with two ungraded school sessions lasting sixteen to twenty weeks each, the medical education system developed a profile that was deficient in many particulars. Certainly, bright, capable, dedicated teachers worked within this structure to produce remarkably brilliant physicians and surgeons. But these successes were achieved in spite of a weakened apprenticeship system, an overreliance on didactic learning, the lack of clinical and demonstrative teaching, lax licensing requirements, and a competitive spirit that matriculated students with little regard to their qualifications or competence.

Perhaps too much has been said in criticism of the early separation of medical schools from the university. Unlike their European counterparts, American universities were devoted principally to instruction in the classics, mathematics, and philosophy and had little connection with professional schools. Indeed, until the introduction of laboratory science into the medical school curriculum, there was little substantive advantage in integrating the medical school into the university. Besides, the rapid expansion of the frontier after 1800 demanded the training of large numbers of practitioners and this need was efficiently and effectively accomplished through the ingenious combination of apprenticeship and proprietary medical schools. Admittedly, the requirements for admission to these schools were minimal, but they produced a cadre of physicians who, while lacking in depth of scientific knowledge, provided a modicum of health care to the sprawling young republic.

For those young men who could afford the expense, Paris became the mecca for modern scientific medicine. There, enterprising young men sought practical training, learned the statistical and analytical study of disease, and, in the process, repaired many of the deficiencies of their didactic education. Postgraduate medical study took on new meaning as Pierre Louis (1787–1872) and other clinical teachers demonstrated the possibility of disease identification on the basis of extensive clinical and postmortem examinations. While short on experimental research, the Paris school of medicine represented a triumph of medical empiricism over metaphysical concepts of disease that had reigned unchallenged for centuries.[13]

To add to the challenge of maintaining medical standards, various state legislatures abandoned their meager licensing regulations that, when combined with the overseeing efforts of medical societies and university governing boards, had ensured some degree of regulatory control over the profession. The reasons for this shift are several, but, in the main, they reflected the egalitarian nature of American culture and its aversion to monopoly, elitism, intellectualism, and restraint of trade. The spirit of democracy ran high as legislatures chose to see little difference between proprietary and university-affiliated medical schools, between regular and irregular practitioners, and between the claims of one medical system and another. In rapid succession, states repealed what medical legislation existed: Illinois in 1826; Ohio in 1833; Mississippi in 1834; the District of Columbia, Maryland, Massachusetts, Maine, Connecticut, and South Carolina in 1838; New York in 1844; Texas in 1848; and Michigan in 1851. By the time of the Civil War, no effective medical licensing existed in any of the states.[14]

Within this tumultuous new medical democracy, Cincinnatians had their pick of several different therapeutic systems. In addition to regular doctors, the city attracted all kinds of medical sectarians, providing a home for herb and Indian doctors, Thomsonians, eclectics, physio-medicalists, and the earliest homeopaths in the Midwest.[15] The editors of the *Medical Observer* of Cincinnati noted in 1857 that "it has become fashionable to speak of the Medical Profession as a body of jealous, quarrelsome men, whose chief delight is the annoyance and ridicule of each other."[16] According to Abraham Flexner, all medicine prior to that which was scientifically based, was sectarian: "Every one started with some sort of preconceived notion; and from a logical point of view, one preconception is as good as another."[17] Essentially, what each therapeutic system—including orthodoxy—viewed as "correct" medicine was simply a relic of extinct science that had acquired the pretense of dogma. In all, seventeen medical schools formed in Cincinnati during the nineteenth century.

ALLOPATHY

Those doctors who boasted an uninterrupted link with the past and decried the undisciplined and iconoclastic efforts of reformers were little better in their views than those they opposed. Known as *old-school*, *regular*, or *allopathic* (from *alloion*, meaning *different*) physicians, they turned to remedies whose effects differed from, but were not directly opposite to, the disease. Drawing upon a rationalistic system founded on the Hippocratic and Galenic supposition that the proper regulation of the body's secretions ensured health, allopathic physicians bled, puked, purged, blistered, and perspired patients as the best means of cure. Using their political clout, they gained control over most municipal hospitals, county and state societies, and boards of examiners, thereby controlling the portals of access and professional legitimacy.

The first regular medical school in Cincinnati was the Medical College of Ohio, chartered through the efforts of Daniel Drake in 1819. As the creative force behind the college, Drake became its first president, while colleagues Coleman Rogers became vice president and Elijah Slack registrar and treasurer. Faculty included Drake as chair of institutes and practice of medicine, Slack in chemistry, Rogers and Jesse Smith in anatomy and surgery, and Benjamin S. Bohrer in materia medica and pharmacy. Medical jurisprudence was divided among the professors, and, after the regular session ended, the college offered a special course of botanical lectures to illustrate the importance of medical botany.[18] Students paid a fee of twenty dollars to attend each professor's lectures; five-dollar fees for matriculation, library, and hospital privileges; and a three-dollar graduation fee to each professor.[19]

Following the second commencement exercises on March 4, 1822, the school erupted in dissension. Not surprisingly, Drake was the spark that ignited most of the school's early disputes, leaving and returning several times, in the course of which he founded several other medical colleges and filled eleven chairs in six different institutions. In comparison to its rival school at Lexington, whose classes averaged 188 over a sixteen-year period, the Cincinnati college matriculated an average of sixty-three per class over the same period. Charged by the legislature with inefficiency, the faculty indignantly responded that they had been distracted by feuds. This admission proved to be one of the understatements of Cincinnati's early medical history.[20]

In its first year of operation, college lectures were held in quarters above a general store owned by Drake's father on 91 Main Street, while its anatomical demonstrations and surgical operations were carried out at the newly organized Commercial Hospital.[21] From 1824 to 1826, the college held classes in a room formerly occupied by the Miami Exporting Company on Front Street near Sycamore before relocating on Sixth Street, between Vine and Race, where it occupied a two-story building containing living quarters in the basement for the janitor and his family; a lecture hall, chemical department, library, and trustees' room on the first floor; and faculty offices, anatomical theater, and various cabinets of teaching materials on the second floor.[22]

In 1851, the college began construction of a four-story Gothic-style building that combined brick and cast iron, painted in imitation free stone. The first floor on each side of the front entrance contained rented store space, with a library, a general lecture room, and two laboratory rooms situated in the rear. The second floor housed six offices rented to physicians and other professionals, along with a museum. On the third floor were offices for four professors and an anatomical lecture room, while the fourth story consisted of six dissecting rooms, an office for the professor of anatomy, a lecture room, and a circular amphitheater.[23] According to John P. Foot in his *Schools of Cincinnati* (1855), "the internal arrangements furnish accommodations for professors and pupils which are said . . . to be unsurpassed, in extent of convenience, by any institution of the kind in the United States."[24]

By midcentury, the college library had nearly two thousand volumes purchased by the state; anatomical cabinets containing skeletons as well as wooden and wax models of more delicate structures; an extensive collection of foreign and domestic animal skeletons; five hundred specimens of diseased bones; a large collection of indigenous plants and their extracts, along with other medicinal preparations used in practice; and various wax casts of women and children for the teaching of obstetrics. Students had access to the Commercial Hospital, where they could observe the medical and surgical treatment of patients by college faculty. By this time, too, the faculty included H. W. Baxley in anatomy, John Locke in chemistry and pharmacy, L. M. Lawson in physiology and pathology, T. O. Edwards in materia medica and therapeutics and medical jurisprudence, Reuben D. Mussey in surgery, Landon C. Rives in obstetrics and the diseases of women and children, John Bell in theory and practice, and John Davis in anatomy. L. M. Lawson also served as dean of the college.[25]

Merged with Cincinnati Medical College (1834) in 1846 and with Miami Medical College from 1857 to 1865, it became the Medical Department of the University of Cincinnati in 1896, and in 1909 it merged with Miami Medical College once again to form the Ohio-Miami Medical College of the University of Cincinnati.[26]

Disappointed in having been voted out by his own faculty, Daniel Drake organized the medical department of Cincinnati College in a two-story brick building on Fourth Street between Main and Walnut. Its founding in 1834 was in response to the alleged poor condition of the Medical College of Ohio and the desire that the state not lose a strong medical institution. Faculty consisted of Drake in theory and practice; Joseph Nash McDowell (nephew of Ephraim McDowell) in special and surgical anatomy; Samuel D. Gross in general and pathological anatomy, physiology, and medical jurisprudence; Horatio G. Jameson and Willard Parker in surgery; Landon C. Rives in obstetrics and diseases of women and children; James B. Rogers and

John L. Riddle in chemistry and pharmacy; and John P. Harrison in materia medica. Despite auspicious beginnings, including a stellar faculty, the institution was short lived. Lack of monies to support the college's equipment and library, exclusion by the faculty of the Medical College of Ohio from access to Commercial Hospital, and the resignation of several of its key faculty led to its dissolution. The department matriculated about four hundred students before merging in 1846 with the Medical College of Ohio.[27]

In 1851, the Cincinnati College of Medicine and Surgery organized under the ambitious leadership of Alvah H. Baker, with the first class graduating in 1852. Classes were first held in a rented building at the corner of Longworth and Western Row that also housed the Marine Hospital and Invalid's Retreat. In 1872, it moved to 164 George Street and, in 1893, to Vine between Liberty and Green. Professors included Baker in surgery; Benjamin S. Lawson, professor of practice; R. A. Spencer, anatomy; Elijah Slack and Charles W. Wright, chemistry; James Graham, materia medica; J. Sidney Skinner, pathology; and Edward Mead, obstetrics and diseases of women and children. The last class graduated in 1902. Its department for women became the Women's Medical College of Cincinnati in 1887 and, later, the Laura Memorial Woman's Medical College, which closed in 1903.[28]

The Miami Medical College, a proprietary college under the leadership of surgeon Reuben D. Mussey, a disgruntled member of the Medical College of Ohio faculty, organized in 1852 and occupied a building on Fifth Street and Central Avenue. Its faculty included Mussey, surgery; Jesse P. Judkins, surgical anatomy and pathology; Charles L. Avery, descriptive anatomy; John Davis, anatomy; John F. White, practice; George Mendenhall, obstetrics and diseases of women and children; John A. Murphy, materia medica, therapeutics, and jurisprudence; C. G. Comegys, institutes of medicine; and H. E. Foote, chemistry. Denied access to Commercial Hospital, students had to rely on the clinical lectures of their professors at St. John's Hotel for Invalids at Third and Plum and a small dispensary attached to the college. Classes graduated from 1853 to 1857, when it merged with the Medical College of Ohio.[29]

In 1865, the school was revived around the leadership of Jesse Judkins, J. A. Murphy, and George Mendenhall and began classes at the Ohio Dental College on College Street before moving in 1866 to permanent quarters on Twelfth near Plum. By 1872, the college was graduating nearly seventy students. It passed out of existence following the 1908–9 session, absorbed into the Ohio-Miami Medical Department of the University of Cincinnati.[30]

HOMEOPATHY

Homeopathy (from *homios*, meaning *like*), was introduced by the German physician Samuel Christian Friedrich Hahnemann (1755–1843), who taught the doctrine of *similia similibus curantur* or, like cures like—a discovery he believed rivaled the significance of Newton's law of gravitation. While translating Cullen's *Treatise on the Materia Medica* into German in 1796, Hahnemann took exception to the author's discussion of the antipyretic virtues of Peruvian bark (cinchona) and began a series of experiments on himself. He soon observed that the bark, which acted as a specific in ague, produced symptoms of intermittent fever. Surprised by the results, he concluded that a true drug possessed the power of causing in healthy persons the same symptoms it cured in the sick. This meant testing each potential drug on a healthy person to determine its pathological effects. Once these effects were understood, it was then possible to prescribe for the sick. Subsequent experiments with belladonna produced a sore throat like that evidenced in scarlet fever and mercury produced symptoms that resembled syphilis. Hahnemann's *Organon der Rationellen Heilkunde*, published in 1810, became the basis of his homeopathic system of disease, a system that won a substantial following in the United States.[31]

What incurred the wrath of old-school doctors was not so much Hahnemann's belief that a spiritual and dynamic disturbance in life brought about a change in health, but that infinitesimal doses of drugs were best suited to treat this immaterial change.[32] In explaining this phenomenon, Hahnemann hypothesized that the manner in which he prepared his medicines added to their medicinal potency—that is, that shaking the drug produced a potentization in which the particles changed from a crude to a dynamic curative force. Thus, small doses of drugs could replace the moderate to heroic doses of mercury, arsenic, and tartar emetic that had become the mainstay of regular practice as well as such traditional medical procedures as cupping, leeching, blistering, counter-irritation, liniments, fomentations, poultices, and ointments. Now a thirteenth dilution of pulsatilla could substitute for the most violent emetic.[33]

Hahnemann's claims were welcomed by converts in America. German immigrants brought his ideas to Northampton County in Pennsylvania, and Hans Burch Gram (1786–1840), an American of Danish extraction, set up practice in New York. Other early converts included John F. Gray, Abraham D. Wilson, A. Gerald Hull, William Channing, Henry Detwiller, and Constantine Herring, often called the father of American homeopathy. Dr. Storm Rosa, who held a position at the Eclectic Medical Institute in Cincinnati, became the first homeopathic teacher in the West. Poet Henry Wadsworth Longfellow, novelist Nathaniel Hawthorne, suffragette Julia Ward Howe, and author Louisa May Alcott followed homeopathic regimens. Homeopathy also claimed among its adherents statesmen Daniel Webster and William Seward and oil magnate John D. Rockefeller.

Cincinnati was home to Pulte Medical College, named after Joseph H. Pulte, a leading homeopath in the city. Organized in 1872, it graduated the first class in 1873. College facilities were located at Seventh and Mound Streets, housing a faculty of nine professors, two lecturers, and one demonstrator of anatomy. Through its large free dispensary, the college focused much of its attention on clinical teaching, which covered nineteen of its thirty-nine weekly lectures. A dedicated board of trustees served the college and its influence was such that the college seldom lacked for resources, being sustained by area businessmen and friends of homeopathy who supported its philosophy of therapeutics. Women were taught separately in some of the branches. In 1910, Pulte merged with the Cleveland Homeopathic Medical College, forming the Cleveland-Pulte Medical College. Classes graduated each year until 1914, when the school and its property transferred to Ohio State University in Columbus and became the Ohio State University College of Homeopathic Medicine.[34]

BOTANICS

As old-school medicine began losing its favored position in the 1820s and 1830s, in part because of its own self-doubts, groups of botanics were announcing that no medical system had a monopoly on truth or practice. Braced by an almost chiliastic belief in the ability of the common man to sort out his own needs, the botanics successfully lobbied state legislatures to nullify the few remaining licensing restrictions. The American dislike for monopoly and its distrust of learned expertise played into the hands of the botanics. Identifying themselves as "reformed" or "new-school" physicians, they sought a radical simplification of Galen and the medical ancients. Here, within popular democracy, lay the basis of an inborn, folk wisdom that overshadowed all of the ratiocinations of orthodoxy. Teaching that God had provided each region of the world with its own medicines, and that the medicinal properties of native plants far excelled any expensive mineral or plant drugs from the Old World, the botanics set about to demonstrate the superiority of their therapeutic practices.[35]

Samuel Thomson (1769–1843), the botanic crusader of the earlier nineteenth century who railed against the heroic remedies of the more fashionable regulars, employed no less harsh medicine in his sheet anchor of lobelia, or emetic herb. His therapeutic system, which he organized in 1805 around successful salesmanship and a network of Friendly Botanic Societies, spread through the Northeast, South, and Midwest with a vigor that rivaled the spread of religious revivalism in the early nineteenth century.

Little of Thomson's theory was new. Having acquainted himself with the names and uses of various roots and herbs as a youth, and learning firsthand how to treat disease from local root doctors, he obtained patent rights for a healing technique that looked and acted surprisingly like Galen's humoral pathology. Thomson attributed disease to the lessening of heat due to an imbalance of the body's humors. With his patented six-step therapeutic regimen of steam and puke, he cleansed and scoured the stomach and bowels, corrected digestion, and restored the body to its proper balance. Lobelia, red pepper, ginger, bayberry, squaw weed, bitterroot, and root of marsh rosemary represented but a few of the seventy plants that became the mainstays of his materia medica.[36]

What began as a protest against the heroic practices of regular medicine turned into a mass movement that swept through the back roads of rural and small-town America. The particular strength of Thomson's system was its democratic appeal. Persons willing to pay twenty dollars could purchase the right to cure themselves and their families of disease and illness without having to rely on the pretensions of a learned professional. Here was a self-help, do-it-yourself system of therapeutic cure open to men and women alike. Soon, agents were spreading Thomson's botanic message and selling rights to his family practice throughout the South and Midwest. In Mississippi, the governor of the state estimated half of its citizens relied on Thomsonism, and in Ohio Thomson's herbal medicines were used by nearly a third of the population.[37]

The principles advocated in Thomson's *New Guide to Health and Botanic Family Physician* (1822), especially the idea of nonpoisonous medication, appealed to many Americans who had tired of orthodoxy's reliance on depletive drugs. Support also came from Harvard physician Benjamin Waterhouse (1754–1846); Yale physician William Tully (1755–1859), compiler of the *Materia Medica, or Pharmacology and Therapeutics* (1857–58); and abolitionist William Lloyd Garrison (1805–1879). Thomson's frequent reference to the writings of Scottish physician William Buchan (1729–1805) and founder of methodism John Wesley (1703–1791), and their desire to demystify medicine, had instant appeal among readers. Moreover, Thomson's stories and anecdotes were crafted to illustrate the common habits of farmers, mechanics, and housewives. While his advice was unexceptional, it carried a common-sense application that glorified self-sufficiency and encouraged families to provide for their own basic medical needs.[38]

The backbone of Thomson's system were his agents, who, like Methodist circuit riders, carried his simple medical system into the heartland of America. In their enthusiasm for selling patents, they became outspoken advocates of Thomsonism, questioning the assumptions of regular medicine and challenging as well the professional class of more educated physicians. But not all of Thomson's agents were true believers. Some were entrepreneurs interested only in their commission, who took license with the patented system in order to augment sales. Others saw in his network of agents a powerful and popular system of practice and concluded that Thomson need not be the *only* provider of common-sense medicine. Still others realized that, despite Thomson's good intentions, botanic medicine promised more than his exclusive patent rights could deliver. The future of botanic medicine, they argued, depended on new leadership and more structured organizations, including botanic infirmaries and medical colleges to ensure the future of reform medical practice.[39]

The Thomsonian movement peaked in the 1840s, riding the crest of other reform efforts that washed over the American landscape. Yet, at the height of the movement, large sections of society, particularly in New England, the South, and the West had adopted the doctrines of botanic medicine. Representative of its success were the activities of hundreds of Friendly Botanic Societies; the founding of more than seventy botanic journals; the establishment of numerous infirmaries and medical schools based on botanic principles; the activities of hundreds of general and local agents and retailers selling patent rights, books, and medicines; and the sympathetic support from the American protestant ministry.[40]

The Physio-Medicals, a formal school of botanic medicine drawn from dissident independent Thomsonians, owed their existence to Alva Curtis (1797–1881), whose bookish approach to medical reform lacked Thomson's grass-roots ties to democracy and the common man. Curtis appealed to the memory of Thomson but pursued a course of medical reform that resulted in the opening of the Botanico-Medical College and Infirmary in April 1836 in Columbus, Ohio. Three years later, he founded the Literary and Botanico-Medical Institute of Ohio, the first state-chartered medical school based on the ideas of the Thomsonian schismatics. In 1841, Curtis moved the school to Cincinnati, where, over a period of ten years, it changed names frequently until taking the name Physio-Medical College, which it retained until closing in 1880. First housed at Madame Trollope's Bazaar on Third, east of Broadway, the college moved several times before finally locating at the Corry Homestead on Auburn Avenue.[41]

From 1836 until 1911, when the last physio-medical school closed in Chicago, thirteen colleges were founded on a high-brow formulation of Thomsonian medicine. Instruction in these colleges followed the principle of aiding the body's vital force by using no deleterious agents. The physios believed that vital force, not the physician, healed disease. This meant aiding the *vis medicatrix naturae,* or the healing power of nature, not hindering it by the use of depletive drugs and regimens. In choosing their medicines, the physios relied on Thomson's sheet anchor—lobelia, capsicum, and the vapor bath—but deliberately chose to expand the botanic materia medica.[42] The physio-medicals were quick to point out the crudities of the steam and puke system, but they never lost sight of Thomson's basic principles. This meant making their own medicines or purchasing them from wholesale drug firms devoted to Thomson's legacy. Unfortunately, the independent Thomsonians lacked sufficient numbers to sustain a distinctive drug trade, forcing them to rely on the materia medica of other sectarians, especially the eclectics.[43]

In a time when the public judged healers more by their reputations than by their schooling, and the ability to diagnose human ills exceeded the ability to successfully treat them, the physios left behind a respected legacy as primary care providers. Certainly none achieved a national reputation; nevertheless, they served as respected practitioners to an appreciative patient population. Herb cures carried no less credibility in nineteenth-century households and were oftentimes the preferred treatment among rural and small-town inhabitants.[44]

The Eclectics

Separate from the Thomsonians and the physio-medicals were the eclectics (from the Greek *eklego*, meaning *to choose from*), whose botanic system of medicine filled an important void in family practice. The name came from its use by Celsus, Agathinos of Sparta, Archigenes of Syria, Galen, and other medical men who preferred to stand apart from prevailing medical schools by choosing whatever curative measures most benefited their patients. Archigenes, styled the "founder of eclecticism," and his pupil Aretaeus were characterized by the lack of bigotry, choosing their curative agents from among the pneumatic, methodic, and dogmatic sects without adhering to any one particular creed. Although this early sect prospered over seven centuries, it lost ground during the age of the Roman Empire. Later descendants took their place in Germany, Italy, France, and England, but none obtained the importance or duration of these forebearers.

The term "eclectic" seemed to define adequately the nature of this reform philosophy, but Alexander Holmes Baldridge (1795–1874), one of the early pioneers of reform medicine, suggested an alternative, the "American School of Medicine." More expressive of the school's protestant origins, it failed to elicit the same level of support. Nonetheless, individual reformers used the terms "eclectic" and "American School" interchangeably.[45]

American eclecticism had its origins in the first quarter of the nineteenth century in the investigations of Jacob Tidd, a German herb doctor from East Amwell, New Jersey, and his student Wooster Beach (1794–1868) of Trumbull, Connecticut. A graduate of the medical department of the University of New York, Beach parted ways with allopathic medicine by identifying almost exclusively with vegetable

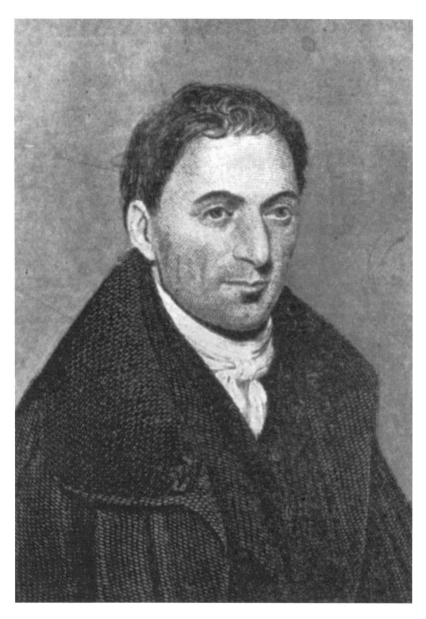

Wooster Beach, M.D. (1794–1868), father of American Reformed Practice. Courtesy of the Lloyd Library and Museum, Cincinnati.

medicines and by being catholic in his selection of the most efficacious principles and agents from all medical systems. Beach was conversant with the botanical literature of his generation, including German physician and botanist Johann David Schoepf (1752–1800); Benjamin Smith Barton's *Elements of Botany* (1803) and his unfinished *Collections for an Essay Towards a Materia Medica of the United States* (1798–1804); Samuel Henry's *A New and Complete American Medical Family Herbal* (1814); Jacob Bigelow's *American Medical Botany* (1817–20); Constantine Samuel Rafinesque's *Medical Flora: Or, Manual of the Medical Botany of the United States of North America* (1828–30); the writings of Robley Dunglison (1798–1869) and William Tully (1785–1859); as well as the United States pharmacopoeias of 1820 and 1830. Having adopted the motto *vires vitales sustinete* (sustain the vital forces), Beach took exception to the practice of bloodletting and the use of strong mineral remedies and moved unhesitatingly toward a more kindly treatment of disease. This he did in opposition to both the Thomsonians and the allopaths.[46]

As part of his crusade to detect the errors of modern practice, Beach began privately instructing students at his New York City home in 1825 and two years later opened a clinical school known as the United States Infirmary. In 1829, he enlarged the school, calling it the Reformed Medical Academy; a year later, it bore the name Reformed Medical College of the City of New York.[47] Assisting him at the college were Thomas Vaughn Morrow, Ichabod Gibson Jones, and John J. Steele, all graduates of regular schools. Each shared Beach's catholic view of botanic medicine and opposed the restrictive and authoritarian views of Samuel Thomson. Beach intended his reformed system of medicine "to release the mind from the dogmas of creeds and systems, the philosophy of medical schools, as they were then taught, and to direct it to an unlimited field of inquiry."[48]

In 1833, Beach published his popular three-volume *American Practice of Medicine*, presenting his views on reformed medicine. The founding principles of his system included admonitions against mercury and other mineral drugs; opposition to salivation and long-continued regimens of depletion; condemnation of bloodletting in all forms; and rejection of unnecessary surgery. Although Beach borrowed extensively from Rafinesque, William P. C. Barton, Jacob Bigelow, and Elisha Smith, his *American Practice of Medicine* became one of the more popular texts of botanical literature in the nineteenth century. His one-volume condensed version (1846) went through fourteen editions and received numerous testimonials and medals of recognition from abroad. Other popular works written by Beach included his *Treatise on Pulmonary Consumption, Phthisis Pulmonalis, with Remarks on Bronchitis* (1840), *Medical and Botanic Dictionary* (1847), and *An Improved System of Midwifery* (1851).[49]

The eclectics were as forcibly opposed to the sweating, vomiting, and enervating regimen of the Thomsonians as they were to the bleeding, blistering, and mercurial purging and salivating regimens of the regulars. Both seemed unsound to eclectic thinking, wedded to obsolete theories of disease and disease nosology. Operating on a parallel but more kindly road to wellness, the eclectics introduced a distinctive pharmacy based on indigenous plant remedies—the resin of podophyllum as a substitute for calomel; betony as an emetic and cathartic; maidenhair for pleurisy and jaundice; compound tar plaster in place of old-school applications of croton oil, cantharides, and tartar emetic; and compound tincture of sanguinaria for emesis.[50] In general, the eclectics favored the natural curative processes of the organism through the use of noninjurious medication; demanded freedom of thought and investigation; supported the development of the vegetable materia medica as the safest method of treating disease; supported the inductive method of investigation; advocated simplicity in prescribing; determined the value of a drug through the treatment of the sick patient rather than through laboratory experimentation; and condemned the extremes of over drugging and therapeutic nihilism.[51]

Throughout their history, the eclectics had an affinity for homeopathy, partly because they found common cause in facing the power and politics of old-school medicine. This affinity also derived from the strength homeopathy claimed among many wealthy and cultured Americans who objected to the "sledgehammer" doses of medicines then in vogue. Equally important, the eclectics were enamored with the homeopath's minimalist approach, believing excessive doses of innocuous drugs retarded the body's natural affinity for self-repair.[52]

Before 1860 thirteen colleges had organized as eclectic or a mixture of eclectic and physio-medical. These included the New York Reformed Medical College (1826–39); College of Medicine, Botanic, in New York City (1836–46); Reformed Medical College of Georgia (1845–61); Eclectic Medical Institute of Cincinnati (1845–1939); Wooster Medical Institute (1846–59); Eclectic Medical Institute of New York (1847–48); Randolph Eclectic Medical Institute (1848–49); Central Medical College of New York (1849–52); Memphis Institute (1849–50); Eclectic Medical College of Pennsylvania (1850–80); Metropolitan Medical College of the City of New York (1853–62); American Medical College (1853–57); and the Cincinnati College of Eclectic Medicine and Surgery (1856–59).

By the end of the century, the eclectics numbered 9,703 compared with 72,028 allopaths, 8,640 homeopaths, and 1,553 physiomedicals.[53] By then, there were eight eclectic colleges, one national and thirty state societies, ten medical journals, and more than sixty medical texts, many of which had become standard works of reference and study. The approved list of eclectic colleges as determined by the national association consisted of the American Medical College at 407 Jefferson Avenue, St. Louis, Missouri (1873); Bennett College of Eclectic Medicine and Surgery at the corner of Ada and Fulton Streets, Chicago, Illinois (1868); California Medical College at 1466 Folsom Street, San Francisco, California (1879); Eclectic Medical College of the City of New York at 239 East 14th Street, New York (1865); Eclectic Medical Institute at 1009 Plum Street, Cincinnati, Ohio (1845); Georgia College of Eclectic Medicine and Surgery at Tanner Street, near Edgewood, Atlanta, Georgia (1886); Lincoln Medical College at 121 South 14th Street, Lincoln, Nebraska (1899); and the American College of Medicine and Surgery, Chicago, Illinois (1901). Together, they formed the National Confederation of Eclectic Medical Colleges.[54] Graduates held positions in private practices, colleges, hospitals, insurance companies, governmental sanitary boards, and as surgeons in the army and navy. Eclectics perceived themselves as an established force in the medical world "and as likely to be permanent as any other doctrine now held in the whole realm of art and science."[55]

After the Council on Medical Education began its classifications of schools, the number of eclectic colleges began to decline. In 1915 there were four schools and after 1920 only one. The Kansas City College of Medicine and Surgery claimed to be eclectic, but it was disowned by the National Eclectic Medical Association as a diploma mill.[56]

Old EMI

Of all the sectarian schools in Cincinnati, none lasted as long or was as popular as the Eclectic Medical Institute. Known affectionately as "Old EMI" by faculty, students, and alumni, it was a proprietary college representing a consolidation of the Worthington Medical College (1830–42), the American Medical College (1853), the Eclectic College of Medicine and Surgery (1857–59), and the Eclectic Medical Institute (1845–1910). The school changed its name to the Eclectic Medical College in 1910 when it reorganized as a not-for-profit educational institution.[57]

EMI had its origins in the Reformed Medical College of Wooster Beach in New York City, which, failing to obtain a charter from the state, looked westward in hope of finding a more agreeable environment. The aspiring village of Worthington, situated in the center of the state on the Whetstone River, nine miles north of Columbus, on the northern turnpike, invited the reformers to join Worthington College, chartered in 1819. While the New York college continued to operate until 1838, its western affiliate opened a medical department in the winter of 1830 with eight students and John J. Steele as president. This was the first sectarian medical school chartered in the United States. Thomas V. Morrow of Kentucky, an ardent abolitionist, known affectionately by students and colleagues as "Old Macrotys" because of his preference for the drug cimicifuga, and also recognized as the "Father of Eclecticism in the West," replaced Steele as dean of the medical faculty and led the young department through its initial years.[58]

For twelve years, the Worthington medical department, located in an oblong two-storied brick building topped by a cupola and bell tower, was the most prominent institution in the practice of reformed medicine in the Midwest. Admission to the medical department required a certificate of good moral character and a good English education. The fall and winter fee schedule in 1834 consisted of anatomy and physiology by T. V. Morrow—twelve dollars; chemistry and medical jurisprudence by G. W. Chevias—twelve dollars; theory and practice of medicine, and midwifery by C. B. Day—ten dollars; surgery and diseases of women and children by Ichabod G. Jones—ten dollars; botany, materia medica, and pharmacy by J. R. Paddock—ten dollars;

fees for each professor's spring and summer course—five dollars; graduation fee—ten dollars; and a dissecting fee (optional)—three dollars.[59] In 1836, the department began publishing a monthly journal, the *Western Medical Reformer*, spelling out the basic principles of reform practice to distinguish its methods from the steam and puke followers of Thomson. By then, nearly two hundred reform practitioners had gone forth from the New York and Worthington schools.[60]

Like any other for-profit institution, the Worthington medical department faced the rigors of the market economy. When the economy was strong, the school did well. Not surprisingly, the financial panic of 1837 left the college in difficult straits and forced the faculty to suspend publication of the journal. More significantly, the town of Worthington was surpassed by other Ohio cities economically. Suffering also from the machinations of allopathic enemies; defections from within its own faculty; strong competition from Alva Curtis and his independent Thomsonians in neighboring Columbus, where they had organized the Botanico-Medical Institute of Ohio; the inability to obtain state appropriations for chemical apparatus, an anatomical museum, and library; and a notorious "resurrection" riot in the autumn of 1839 that destroyed Morrow's home and nearly ended in mob violence against the faculty, the school closed and moved to Cincinnati. There, during the winter of 1842–43, Morrow established temporary accommodations in the Hay Scales House on the corner of Sixth and Vine Streets where students sat through four to six lectures daily and paid fees for a single four-month session amounting to fifty-five dollars.[61]

The earliest faculty at the newly named Reformed Medical School of Cincinnati, Ohio, included Alexander H. Baldridge in obstetrics, diseases of women and children, and surgery; Lorenzo E. Jones in therapeutics, materia medica, pharmacy, and physiology; Thomas Vaughan Morrow in theory and practice of medicine, operative surgery, and anatomy; Benjamin Lord Hill in anatomy; and James Kilbourne, Jr., in materia and therapeutics. Kilbourne died of consumption shortly after his first course of lectures. His father, Colonel James Kilbourne, Sr. had been responsible for inviting the eclectics to Worthington.[62]

Following a successful petition drive of eleven hundred Cincinnatians, including the mayor and members of the city council, and against the vocal opposition of the Ohio Medical College faculty, Morrow and his supporters managed to secure, by a special act of the

Ohio Legislature on March 10, 1845, a charter as the Eclectic Medical Institute of Cincinnati. The bill of incorporation established a board of trustees numbering between eleven and fifteen, chosen by the stock-holders whose votes were based on the number of shares held. The board appointed the faculty, to consist of at least five professors compe-tent to deliver lectures in the area of anatomy, physiology, pathology, materia medica, obstetrics, medical jurisprudence, practice of medi-cine, and surgery.

According to the charter, no student could present himself as a can-didate for graduation unless he was at least twenty-one years of age; of good moral character; regularly engaged in the study of physic and surgery with a respectable practitioner for at least three years (or four in apprenticeship and one course of lectures); had attended two full courses of lectures at a legally incorporated medical college, the last course having been taken at EMI; and passed a "thorough, critical, and impartial examination" prepared by the faculty and including sub-ject matter from each of the departments of medical science.[63] The bill of incorporation also required the college to have a property value of at least ten thousand dollars before diplomas could be granted. This challenge spurred efforts to erect a building on the northwest corner of Court and Plum Streets, which was completed November 7, 1846. Funds for the building at 1009 Plum Street came principally from con-tributions by professors Lorenzo E. Jones, Thomas V. Morrow, Alex-ander H. Baldridge, and Benjamin L. Hill. Wooster Beach, the founder of American eclecticism, was elected to the board of trustees and also taught clinical medicine and surgery.[64]

At the time, the only available text on the "Beachite" style of reform medicine was Beach's own *The American Practice* (1833). Al-though there were a number of works published by the Thomsonians before Beach issued his major work, none were eclectic in principle. Until texts became available from the college's own faculty, students relied on William Barber's *Improved System of Botanical Medical Prac-tice* (1829), Elisha Smith's *Botanic Physician* (1829), and Hervey Whit-ing's *Reformed Practice of Medicine* (1831), in addition to various allo-pathic texts.

In 1846, the school boasted 127 students, exceeding the Medical College of Ohio, the Transylvania Medical School, and the Louisville Medical Institute where Daniel Drake was teaching. By 1855, the col-lege had matriculated 2,145 students and had graduated 593 doctors.[65]

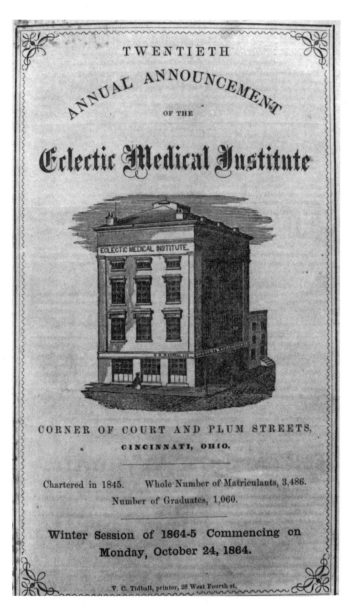

TWENTIETH

ANNUAL ANNOUNCEMENT

OF THE

Eclectic Medical Institute

CORNER OF COURT AND PLUM STREETS,

CINCINNATI, OHIO.

Chartered in 1845.   Whole Number of Matriculants, 3,486.
Number of Graduates, 1,060.

Winter Session of 1864-5 Commencing on
Monday, October 24, 1864.

V. O. Tidball, printer, 28 West Fourth st.

Eclectic Medical Institute, Court and Plum Streets, Cincinnati, erected in 1845. Note the drug manufacturer W. H. Merrell and Company offices on the first floor. Courtesy of the Lloyd Library and Museum.

Indeed, despite external feuds and internal upheavals, the college was a success, enrolling a greater number of students than any other medical school west of the Alleghenies. In an age when both public and medical opinion identified size as an important indicator of quality, the college ranked high among the recognized medical colleges in the country, with 428 matriculants in its first three years, compared with 225 in the medical department of Transylvania University, 404 in Louisville Medical Institute, and 73 in the Medical College of Ohio.[66]

EMI ENROLLMENT DATA

YEARS	MATRICULANTS	GRADUATES
1845–46	81	22
1846–47	127	31
1847–48	220	48
1848–49	191	47
1849–50	224	65
1850–51	211	45
1851–52	212	58
1852–53	308	70
1853–54	292	126
1854–55	279	81

Unlike many less prosperous proprietary schools, EMI offered good facilities, open admission to female students, a Saturday clinic for practical instruction, and a program of instruction comparable in content to most allopathic schools. Its sixteen-week session included seven lectures each day and extra courses in the spring and summer consisting of ten to fifteen lectures each, delivered by the faculty at the request of the class.

By the standards of the trans-Appalachian West, EMI represented the voice of democratic individualism and social criticism that gave to its faculty, students, and alumni a combined sense of optimism and genuine righteousness. They saw themselves blazing new trails through the unknowns of medicine, achieving what their forebears had only dreamed. Opportunistic, they laid claim to every new idea, recounting that their indigeneous American school had broken from Old World orthodoxy and was originating new paths of understanding. They imagined themselves unambiguous progressives and discounted their internal dissensions as simply reflections of their protestant roots and their appetite for self-examination.

CHAPTER TWO

All the Dean's Men

EIGHT DEANS DIRECTED the affairs of the college over the ninety-four years of its existence. By any standard, this formidable statistic demonstrated the stability of the institution despite its spirit of individualism and history of sharp internal disagreements. On the whole, the deanery consisted of skillful politicians who, trusting their own sensibilities, maintained a community of minds amid the perils of medical reform. Thomas Vaughan Morrow (1845–50), Joseph Rodes Buchanan (1850–56), and Robert Safford Newton (1856–61) brought the college through its turbulent years; John Milton Scudder (1861–94) and Frederick J. Locke (1894–1903) provided leadership in the era of the school's renaissance; and Rolla L. Thomas (1904–31), Eben B. Shewman (1934–35), and Byron H. Nellans (1931–33; 1935–39) carried the college through its final years of curricular reorganization, accreditation struggles, and closing.

Equally important to the leadership of the college was its secretary, the only full-time administrator. John K. Scudder, scion of owner John Milton Scudder, held this position from 1888 to 1929. As secretary, Scudder was the chief operating officer and, until the college became a not-for-profit institution in 1909, was chief executive officer as well, responsible to the Scudder family, which owned the majority of shares. Both Frederick J. Locke and Rolla L. Thomas, who served as deans of the faculty during John K. Scudder's years as secretary, were essentially part-time administrators, maintaining private practices and serving principally as spokesmen for the faculty. After Scudder's death in 1929, Byron Nellans became secretary and then, on Shewman's resignation in 1935, assumed the dual role of dean and secretary.

YEARS OF TURBULENCE

The period spanned by the first three deans was marked by contentiousness both within the reform movement itself and between the reform movement and regular medicine. Eclectic reformers considered themselves medical protestants, deliberately casting themselves adrift from the authority of allopathic medicine. As medical iconoclasts, they chafed at the boundaries set by medical orthodoxy and proposed instead that each physician seek authority within his own convictions. Few who stood for and taught eclectic medicine in the early years of medical reform were peacemakers; high-spirited, they drew strength from controversy and rallied around any effort directed at the errors of medical orthodoxy. Reflecting on this early band of reformers, John M. Scudder observed that "they were very warlike, pugnacious as snapping turtles, but they had abundant cause for it; they were Ishmaelites, and every man's hand was against them, and they were inclined to turn their hands against other people."[1]

Among the stalwarts of reform medicine who joined the school in its early years were homeopaths Storm Rosa (1791–1864), Horatio Page Gatchell (1815–1886), and Benjamin L. Hill (1813–1871), the brother-in-law of Thomas Vaughan Morrow; cerebral physiologist and medical philosopher William Byrd Powell (1799–1866); John Milton Sanders, who occupied the chair of chemistry, toxicology, and pharmacy and had once worked in Michael Faraday's laboratory in the Royal Institution of London; distinguished surgeon and teacher Zoheth Freeman (1826–1898); and author and discoverer of the resins and oleoresins John King (1813–1893). These were followed by author, adventurer, and Confederate brigadier general George Washington Lafayette Bickley (1823–1867); author and editor William Sherwood (1812–1871); chemist Daniel Vaughn (d. 1879); teacher, researcher, and later territorial governor of Wyoming John Wesley Hoyt (1831–1912); turbulent and eccentric author Lorenzo E. Jones (1809–1878); author and editor Charles Harley Cleaveland (1820–1863); mathematician, physicist, chemist, judge, and U.S. minister to Italy Johann Bernhard Stallo (1823–1900); and Andrew Jackson Howe (1825–1892), surgeon and opponent of Lister. Most of the faculty were themselves graduates of the institute and at least ten from this early group are included in the *Dictionary of American*

Thomas Vaughan Morrow, M.D.
(1804–1851), founder and president
of EMI (1845–50) and known as
"Father of Eclecticism in the West."
Courtesy of the Lloyd Library
and Museum.

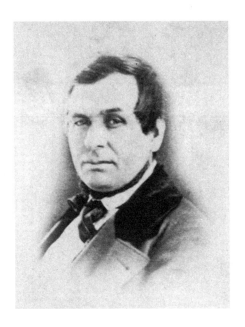

Biography, an indication of their distinction within the medical and
scientific community in pre–Civil War America.[2]

The school's founding dean, Thomas Vaughan Morrow (1804–1851),
the so-called "Father of Eclecticism in the West," grew up in Fairview,
Kentucky. Following his education at Transylvania University in Lexington, he graduated from a regular medical college in New York before
attending the Reformed Medical College of Wooster Beach. Included
in the inner circle of "Beachite" reformers, he soon found himself (all
six feet and 250 pounds) taking over the leadership of the Reformed
Medical College of Ohio, formed in 1830 at Worthington. Morrow,
only twenty-six at the time, worked with the zeal of a true believer,
charting the school's course through the turbulence caused by court
suits, internal dissensions and schisms, a financial panic, and a mob
attack on the college. Following the close of the Worthington medical department, Morrow brought his faculty to Cincinnati, where
in 1842 he organized the Reformed Medical School of Cincinnati
and obtained a charter as the Eclectic Medical Institute. According
to Harvey W. Felter, eclectic medicine's earliest historian, the years

encompassed by Morrow's deanship represented the "formative" period of American reformed medicine.[3]

A successful practitioner as well as dean and professor of theory and practice, Morrow filled the pages of the *Western Medical Reformer* with articles on the principles and practice of reform medicine. Revered by students, he was once described as "a man of rarest talent, a teacher of the greatest success, and a pillar in whose sustaining capacity the Eclectic Medical Institute can confide in all the storms she may encounter from jealousy, envy, or malignity, as she rises to an inestimable position in the work of medical reformation." Following Morrow's death, colleague Ichabod Gibson Jones (d. 1857) brought together his collected writings in a two-volume work titled *The American Eclectic Practice of Medicine* (1853–54).[4]

After Morrow died, the faculty then turned for leadership to the medical philosopher and speculative reasoner Joseph Rodes Buchanan (1814–1899), who graduated from Louisville Medical College in 1842. As a student, he focused on cerebral physiology, becoming a colorful and outspoken lecturer on two new sciences, which he called *psychometry* (demonstrating the influence on the cerebral tissue of one individual by the aura of another) and *sarcognomy* (the sympathetic relations between the parts of the body and the indwelling soul). He also published *The Journal of Man* (1849–56; 1887–90) as a public forum for his ideas and observations. Failing in his effort to bring the two new sciences before the scientific community, Buchanan turned to teaching, occupying the chair of institutes of medicine and diagnosis at the American Medical Institute (Independent Thomsonian) of Cincinnati, which held classes in the Fourth Street Hall. Soon after befriending Morrow in 1846, he joined EMI as professor of physiology and institutes of medicine.

A truculent man, Buchanan bullied his way into the deanship and, until his expulsion in 1856, set a course for the college that included the establishment of a chair of homeopathy, the incorporation of his neurological theories into the curriculum, implementation of a "free education" scheme that nearly bankrupted the college, and participation in feuds and schisms too numerous to count. Believing that strong punitive behavior was the best deterrent to malcontents, Buchanan carried out intemperate attacks on colleagues and students alike. What he lacked in actual medical knowledge, he made up for as ceremonial spokesman for the college. He accepted the privileges and

Joseph Rodes Buchanan (1814–1899),
dean of EMI (1850–56) and editor of
The Eclectic Medical Journal. Courtesy of
the Lloyd Library and Museum.

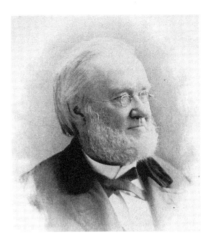

status of his office, embraced irrevocable strategies, and preferred raw
power to pragmatic wisdom or diplomacy. After his expulsion from
EMI for having used tuition dollars for his own personal use and
having participated in a cabal intended to vote in a bogus board of
trustees and issue new stock, he formed with other dissenters a rival
but short-lived Eclectic College of Medicine and Surgery on Walnut
Street, between Fourth and Fifth Streets. He subsequently moved to
Louisville, where he ran unsuccessfully on the Peace platform for the
United States Congress, and then on to New York, where he became
professor of physiology at the Eclectic Medical College of New York
City, and later to Boston, where he opened a College of Therapeutics
to promulgate his idiosyncratic views on physiology, sarcognomy,
psychometry, clairvoyance, and the healing arts. In his latter years,
Buchanan actively resisted the passage of medical licensing laws
and, after moving to California, spent his final years preparing a two-
volume *Primitive Christianity* (1897–98), which represented the full
development of his medical and spiritual beliefs.[5]

The third leader of the college during these early years was
Robert Safford Newton (1818–1881) of Gallia County, Ohio, who attended school at Lewisburg, Virginia, before apprenticing himself to
Dr. Edward Naret of Gallipolis, Ohio, and entering medical school in
Louisville, Kentucky, from which he graduated as a regular physician
in 1841. In 1845, Newton identified with the eclectic school of reform medicine and, in 1849, took the chair of surgery at the Memphis

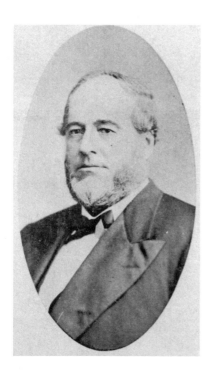

Robert Safford Newton, M.D.
(1818–1881), dean of EMI (1856–61)
and owner of Newton's Clinical Institute.
Courtesy of the Lloyd Library and
Museum.

Institute. There he developed a successful practice until persuaded by a
group of EMI emissaries in 1851 to take the chair of surgery in Cincinnati. The addition of Newton to the faculty brought many positive
changes, including the publication of the *Eclectic Medical Journal*, with
both Newton and Buchanan as co-editors. This journal replaced *The
Western Medical Reformer* founded by Morrow. However, protracted
disagreements and continued fiscal embarrassment plagued the college as long as Buchanan was dean. Fortunately for the college's sake,
Buchanan lacked the resources to purchase the school and was forced
instead to rely on Newton's skills as treasurer to keep it solvent. In
addition to this duty, Newton held the chair of theory and practice and
also conducted Newton's Clinical Institute (replacing Wooster Beach's
clinic) on Sixth and John Streets, affording students optional clinical instruction—that is, observing operations and watching faculty
treat varied and difficult diseases. The clinic charged patients a weekly
rate of from three dollars to seven dollars for room and board and,
while accepting all types of disease, specialized in cancer and fistulous

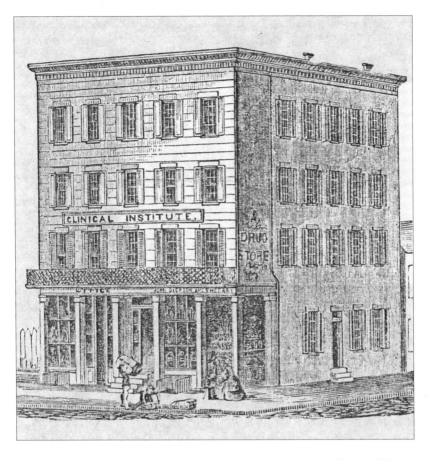

Newton Clinical Institute, Sixth and John Streets, Cincinnati, 1859. Used by EMI students and faculty. Note the John Dickson Apothecary offices on the first floor. Courtesy of the Lloyd Library and Museum.

disorders. The clinic attended to the wants of the most fastidious, with servants in attendance and meals provided at all hours.[6]

For a period of ten years, Newton edited and published the *Eclectic Medical Journal*, assisted in editing the *Eclectic Medical Review* and *Medical Eclectic*, and edited and published numerous books on the materia medica, practice of medicine, surgery, and diseases of children. For a brief two years (1859–60), Newton even managed to take the contents of the *Edinburgh Medical and Surgical Journal* and reissue it under the title of the *Cincinnati Eclectic and Edinburgh Medical Journal*.

He did this believing that, among the medical schools of old world, Edinburgh University manifested the leading liberal and reform channel of ideas and was the most rational representative of medical science abroad. However, according to the editors of the *Cincinnati Lancet and Observer*, the official organ of the city's rival Ohio Medical College, this reissuing was an act of "astonishing impudence" perpetuated on the medical profession by a small group of men "who were never heard of beyond the limits of a small country village" and whose practice consisted of little more than steam, roots, phrenology, homeopathy, and similar humbugs.[7]

After Buchanan's expulsion, Newton became both dean and treasurer, organizing a new faculty, negotiating in 1857 the acquisition of a valuable pathological museum from the defunct American Medical College, and consolidating the institute with rival Eclectic College of Medicine and Surgery in 1859. Now free from internal dissensions and confident of its future, the school focused on expanding its hegemony over reformed medicine in the Midwest. Unanticipated was the emerging crisis of union. With the outbreak of the Civil War, the school faced the prospect of smaller classes, diminished resources, and fear that the city would fall into the hands of the Confederacy.

The war and the resulting diminished income for the college were not the only threats to the school's existence at this time. Reliance on so-called "eclectic concentrations" or "green drugs," which Newton had encouraged, eventually undermined the integrity of the college as well as that of several other reform medical schools that had adopted these drugs. The concentrations were the work of physician John King (1813–1893), identified by eclectics as the father of the reform materia medica, whose *American Dispensatory* (1852) went through eighteen editions and advanced the school beyond crude drugs in powder, infusion, and decoction by introducing the resins of podophyllum and macrotys, which together with the alkaloids of hydrastis and sanguinaria became mainstays of eclectic practice.[8] King's clinical research into the resin of macrotys (cimicifuga racemosa) and the oleoresins of iris, black cohosh, and Culvers root (leptandra) established the therapeutic value of these medicines. The resins and oleoresins represented the medicinal principles of plants precipitated by water from their alcoholic solutions. Prepared by pharmacist William Stanley Merrell (1797–1880) of Cincinnati in the form of extracts or thick oils, these bitter tasting medicines were quickly embraced by eclectic physicians, who designated them concentrated or positive medicines, essential tinctures, or, simply, green drugs.[9]

Reform physicians found it easier to rely on these concentrated solutions than to prepare their own compounds, teas, and decoctions. For several decades, reformers used these medicines as alternatives to the alkaloid pharmaceuticals then being introduced into allopathic medicine and the infinitesimal triturations of homeopathy.[10] By the 1850s, the public had identified eclectic practice with concentrated medicines to a degree that dwarfed all other aspects of its reform philosophy. But as pharmaceutical companies stepped in to profit from the lucrative new industry, few endeavored to ensure that the products issued as eclectic concentrations were worthy of the title. To make matters worse, reform faculty and their medical colleges became embroiled in the competitive struggles of these companies and allegations abounded of adulteration and the lack of scientific investigation. John King, who first introduced these medicines into the eclectic materia medica, denounced the resinoidal craze as a system of medication run wild and withdrew his endorsement except for the few he himself had discovered.[11] He not only condemned concentrated preparations as "a most stupendous fraud," but he also warned fellow reformers that the preparations were tarnishing the cause of eclecticism.[12] Unfortunately, the resinoid trade became identified with reform medicine, particularly eclecticism, and King's worst fears materialized in the closing of a half-dozen eclectic schools as well as several physio-medical colleges that had adopted concentrated medicines into their own botanic systems of practice.

Through the years of the Buchanan and Newton deanships, the college failed to realize much in the way of a "profit" for its stockholders. In 1856, thirty-three stockholders owned 719 shares worth $14,600 in original value.[13] Fortunately for the college, most of the stockholders viewed their shares more as an ideological statement than as a financial investment. In 1860, tuition amounted to $2,939 while the cash expended for salaries and expenses was $1,669.48, leaving a balance of $1,269.52 that the shareholders divided among the faculty.[14] By 1860, receipts from students barely paid for expenses, and the *Eclectic Medical Journal,* which once had a circulation of eighteen hundred subscribers, had diminished to a paltry five hundred, forcing the journal to suspend publication for six months in 1861. In that same year, the cash received from tuition amounted to $854, a situation due

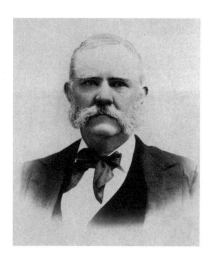

John Milton Scudder (1829–1894), owner, dean, and treasurer of EMI (1861–94). Courtesy of the Lloyd Library and Museum.

principally to the Civil War. Of that amount, $712.29 went toward salaries and expenses, leaving a profit of $141.71, or $23.61 to each member of the faculty.[15] The institute was mortgaged for nearly its actual worth and had to forgo publishing its annual announcement in the winter of 1861 in order to purchase coal.[16]

Scudder Years

Not until John Milton Scudder (1829–1894) assumed control of the college was there some measure of assurance for reform medicine. Born in Harrison, Ohio, young Scudder began work in a button factory at the age of ten. A few years later, he entered Miami University at Oxford, Ohio, after which he became a cabinetmaker and painter. He joined the Swedenborgian Church and, in 1849, married Jane Hannah, with whom he had five children. The deaths of three of his children prompted an interest in medicine, and he selected eclectic physician Milton L. Thomas as his preceptor. In 1856, at the age of twenty-six, he graduated as valedictorian from EMI and immediately joined the faculty as professor of anatomy. Later, he filled the chairs of obstetrics and diseases of women and children and pathology and practice of medicine. He also formed a successful partnership with Orin E. Newton, M.D., and built a strong medical practice in the Fulton section of Cincinnati. In 1861, after the death of his wife,

Scudder married Mary Hannah, the sister of his first wife. With her he also had five children.[17]

In addition to building one of the more lucrative practices in the city, Scudder invested heavily in land in Avondale, a suburb of Cincinnati. The success of these investments enabled him to acquire the majority shares of EMI stock at a time when the school was in financial ruins, the stockholders were despondent over its future, and the journal was reduced in subscriptions. In saving the charter and preventing discredit to its graduates, Scudder earned the respect of King, Howe, Freeman, and other key members of the faculty. Equally significant, from the time Scudder took over ownership of the school, there was no jealousy, schism, or quarrels among the members of the faculty. According to Zoheth Freeman, "From the day he took hold of the Institute every debt was paid; every professor received his recompense promptly; and no worthless notes reflecting on the profession were floating about. Thrift, comfort, peace and good credit came to those who were discouraged and despondent, and Eclecticism became a power in the land."[18]

As owner, dean, and treasurer, Scudder instituted strict management principles to resolve the school's financial embarrassment. He purchased and then revived the school's medical journal, hired a new cohort of dedicated faculty, and steered the institution on a course of fiscal stability. A prolific writer, Scudder added numerous works to the canon of eclecticana and used the pages of the journal to spread information on eclecticism in general and the college in particular. By the late 1860s, the college touted the largest classes of any medical school in the United States, averaging 187 graduates each year.[19]

Scudder brought peace to the institute by paying professors promptly for their services and relieving them of the responsibility for student admissions and other administrative activities. Essentially, he encouraged the faculty to attend to their own private practices, which he felt were far more important for the future of eclecticism than consuming their energies in the school's internal affairs. For their part, the faculty consented to Scudder's personal leadership, satisfied that he served the interest of reformed medicine. This relationship was best exemplified in the faculty's willingness to follow Scudder as he gradually changed the direction of eclectic therapeutics by introducing the concept of specific disease and specific medication. For thirty years, his editorial columns recorded the slow but perceptible change in direction that he brought to eclecticism. No eclectic author was better known.[20]

The beginning years of Scudder's deanship represented a time of change across the medical landscape. For one thing, regular physicians who bled, purged, blistered, puked, perspired, and salivated their patients became the exception to medical practice. About all that remained of heroic practice were cantharides plasters and croton-oil vesicants. By then, too, the Thomsonian movement had all but disappeared and, in its place, independent or reform Thomsonians (better known as "physios" or "physio-medicals") were substituting less drastic botanicals for the harsher steam and puke regimens of earlier years. Not surprisingly, the eclectics, under Scudder's leadership, moved aggressively away from their foul-tasting compounds and concentrated medicines.[21] With the public's loss of faith in these remedies, Scudder observed that EMI had been badly demoralized by its connection with them: "We reached the lowest ebb about 1861 . . . when it did seem as if our school would be merged into the others, a portion going back to the old school and a portion going to the Homeopaths. . . . We were overweighed with men who, whilst claiming to be Eclectics, talked and acted something else."[22]

The eclectics viewed the thirty-year period from roughly 1870 to 1900 as their renaissance. The fire that destroyed the roof, library, and fourth floor of the college on November 20, 1869, was a blessing in disguise, since, for many supporters of eclecticism, the dedication ceremonies marking its replacement represented a rebirth of the American school of reform medicine. The trustees authorized the erection of the building at 228 Court Street adjoining the old building on the north and fronting on Plum Street. Entrance to the college was by a flight of stone steps under a Corinthian portico eighteen feet high, with a doorway eight feet wide by fifteen feet high. Inside on the second floor, a hall thirty-by-seventy feet could seat three hundred. On the first floor were faculty and chemistry rooms, urinals, and waterclosets. The third floor contained an amphitheater thirty-by-seventy feet with a twenty-foot ceiling and seats arranged in a half circle. It was lighted front and rear and by a large skylight over the anatomist's table. The fourth floor housed the dissecting room, fitted with holding tanks and washing tables. At the rear of the building, on the top floor, was a hatchway with a hoisting wheel used to lift cadavers from wagons

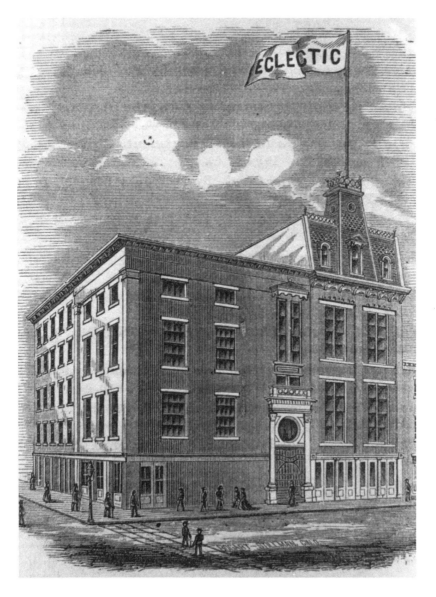

Eclectic Medical Institute, Court and Plum Streets, Cincinnati, 1883. Courtesy of the Lloyd Library and Museum.

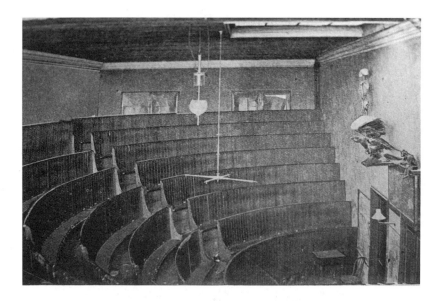

EMI amphitheater, ca. 1885. Courtesy of the Lloyd Library and Museum.

driven through the alley. And mounted on the roof was a turret from which an "Eclectic" banner waved. More than three hundred physicians from across the country celebrated the building's dedication in 1871.[23]

In 1869 Scudder introduced the concept of specific medication, which eventually became the watchword of modern eclecticism and the principal therapeutic doctrine taught in varying degrees at all eclectic colleges. Although specific medication had been practiced by homeopaths for many decades, Scudder claimed to have placed it on a more precise theoretical and practical foundation.[24] "Well do I remember the day when Dr. John M. Scudder entered the business house of H. M. Merrell and Co., with the manuscript of *Specific Medication* balanced in the palm of his hand," recalled pharmacist and eclectic John Uri Lloyd. Scudder reportedly remarked: "This book will either make, or break, the Eclectic school of medicine."[25] To the astute observer, specific medication represented an alliance struck between Scudder and the pharmaceutical firm of H. M. Merrell and Company (later to be Lloyd Brothers, Pharmacists, Inc.).[26]

Having copyrighted the labels of his specific medicines, Scudder ensured quality control by turning the manufacture of the medicines over to Merrell. In this way, he avoided the problems that had plagued King's positive medicines and concentrations. According to Lloyd, Scudder was a true eclectic, seeking in the materia medicas of the homeopath, Thomsonian, physio-medical, and regular any and all simple remedies to replace the depletive medicines of earlier times. As a borrower from other systems, Scudder was thought by some to be a "pseudo-homeopath" since his doses were small and intended for therapeutic action and not physiological shock. Nevertheless, he continued to draw from the American materia medica of John David Schoepf, Benjamin Smith Barton, James Thacher, and Wooster Beach. By inaugurating a series of clinical therapeutic investigations more systematic than anything eclectics had previously attempted, Scudder further refined drug applicability while abandoning many less valuable agents, including the faddish use of resinoids.[27]

The theory of specific medication assumed that disease manifested itself by certain well-defined symptoms and that the totality of symptoms expressed a condition to which a special disease name was given. But the disease name was of value only in the study of the natural history of diseases, for statistical data, or for establishing a prognosis, *not* as a guide for treatment. In treating a patient, the eclectic physician first identified the conditions or symptoms that revealed the disease. Following identification, the eclectic prescribed specific remedies for the specific conditions. In other words, the eclectic held that a fixed relationship existed between drug force and disease expression. There was no law of cure, only empiricism and experimentation centered on the successful employment of a remedy for a particular condition.[28]

In his role as dean, owner, and treasurer of the college, Scudder avoided the trap of conceptualizing the academic enterprise in the abstract, not wanting or having the curiosity to know its particulars. He was the type of administrator who regarded his office as serving an enterprise larger than himself. Although he had little wish to punish opponents or critics, he did not avoid tough issues, being tested early and often as he attempted to replace older faculty with younger and more vigorous teachers. When Scudder received complaints from faculty and students that the lectures of professor Lorenzo E. Jones were outdated, he attempted to arrange a mutually agreeable retirement.

When Jones refused even to consider Scudder's gentle prodding, the trustees stepped in and removed Jones from the faculty. Jones sued, alleging that his professorship was in perpetuity, but the Superior Court of Cincinnati upheld the action of the trustees.[29]

Scudder's long tenure as dean gave him the unique opportunity to change the quality and character of the school through his appointments to the faculty. By the 1880s and 1890s, many of the old stalwarts of reform medicine had either passed from the scene or were reaching retirement. Rather than reach out to many younger doctors who had taken postdoctoral work in Germany, Scudder chose to hire the school's own graduates. Exemplary of this, three out of the four faculty who held chairs in anatomy during this period had graduated from EMI. The same applied to two of the three who taught physiology; one of three in chemistry, pharmacy, and toxicology; both doctors who taught theory and practice of medicine; three out of four teachers of surgery; the single chair in materia medica and therapeutics; one of the two faculty in obstetrics and diseases of women and children; all four who taught physical diagnosis, hygiene, and electricity; all three demonstrators of anatomy; both instructors of clinical medicine; and one of the two in clinical surgery and operative gynecology.

Under Scudder's skillful leadership, EMI grew in stature, becoming the leading eclectic college in the country and the ideological center for medical reform thinking. Eighteen faculty texts graced the shelves of the school's library and, aided by Scudder's theories on specific medication, eclectic thinking went through a resurgence among the remaining schools dedicated to the principles of eclecticism. Beginning with his rehabilitation of the *Eclectic Medical Journal*, his *Eclectic Medical Practice* (1864), *Principles of Medicine* (1869), and *Specific Medication and Specific Medicines* (1870), Scudder led the college into its best years.

Scudder made every effort to ensure that EMI remained in the forefront of eclectic theory. He viewed every other eclectic college as an offspring of the "Mother College" and took pride in their successes. Equally important, he showed resolute opposition to those schools that could not keep pace or that lacked sufficient monetary backing. Such institutions were as much a threat to the good of eclecticism as they were to the education of their students.[30]

Gradually, Scudder was forced by age and infirmities to relinquish some of his duties. First, he turned his lectures over to Rolla Thomas, who trained under his supervision. Later, he turned the business side of the college over to his son, John K. Scudder, who possessed many of the managerial traits of his father.

Finally, it is important to point out two other faculty who dominated the Scudder era: John King, who, as noted earlier, developed the eclectic materia medica; and Andrew Jackson Howe, who perfected eclectic surgery. Along with Scudder, they were known as the "Eclectic Trinity." Together, this threesome steered the school into its renaissance years.[31] John King, a graduate of the Reformed Medical College of Wooster Beach in 1838, located his practice first in New Bedford, Massachusetts, but moved in 1846 to Kentucky, becoming close friends with the Worthington reformers. He was one of the founding members of the National Eclectic Medical Association and held a position at the eclectic school in Memphis until invited to take the chair of obstetrics and diseases of women and children at EMI, a position he held from 1851 to 1890. During his long tenure, he did much to clarify eclectic practice. Students at the college referred to him as "Pappy King."[32] The third member of the trinity, Andrew Jackson Howe, was the best-known eclectic surgeon in the United States. A graduate of Harvard College (1853), Jefferson Medical College (1854), and Wooster Medical Institute (1855), he joined the Cincinnati school in 1857 and held the chair of surgery from 1861 until his death in 1892. A critic of aseptic methods, he nonetheless made a reputation as a bold surgeon and a medico-legal expert. His writings included *A Treatise of Fractures and Dislocations* (1873), *Manual of Eye Surgery* (1874), *Art and Science of Surgery* (1876), and *Operative Gynecology* (1890).[33]

CONSOLIDATION YEARS

With the death of John M. Scudder on February 17, 1894, his shares of stock were divided among his sons—John King Scudder (400), who had assumed managerial control of the college seven years prior to the death of his father; Paul R. Scudder (250), a graduate of the Ohio College of Dental Surgery and manager of his father's estate; Henry Ford Scudder (175), a graduate of EMI in 1893, who eventually moved his practice to California; and William Byrd Scudder (175), an 1890 graduate of EMI and a specialist in eye and ear diseases. Annual stock-holder meetings typically consisted of a gathering of the brothers in the college office, with Henry Ford Scudder sitting as chair and John K. Scudder as secretary. Their business consisted of electing trustees for the ensuing year, followed by a treasurer's report. In 1903, for ex-ample, gross receipts for the college amounted to $9,368.55, of which $8,143.87 went toward expenses, leaving $1,224.68 in gross profits. In this instance, the brothers voted to pay John K. Scudder the profits to cover office expenses as well as his salary as secretary to the college and general manager of the Scudder Brothers Corporation.[34]

In 1894, the brothers appointed as dean Frederick J. Locke (1829–1903), a decided favorite among the students. Born in England and educated at Christ's College, he read medicine with a Dr. Edwards before emigrating to America at the age of seventeen. In 1864, he graduated from EMI and returned in 1871, where, in addition to hold-ing a chair in materia medica and therapeutics, he collaborated with Harvey Wickes Felter in publishing *Locke's Syllabus of the Eclectic Materia Medica and Therapeutics*. A quiet and unassuming teacher, he practiced medicine for more than forty years at 190 Monmouth Street in Newport, Kentucky, and taught for nearly twenty-five. Earnest, yet easygoing, he "never tried to flaunt his superiority or to puzzle anybody by asking intricate questions." He gave four lectures each week on the general principles of drug action, the methods of proving medicinal substances, and the specific effects produced by drugs in various dis-eases. Locke's most popular lecture was on "Sense and Non-Sense in Medicine," which he gave each year to a packed auditorium.[35]

Following in the footsteps of his predecessor, Locke and manager John K. Scudder continued the practice of hiring graduates of the college as faculty. Of the twenty-three faculty and clinical positions in the college in 1901, only five were not EMI graduates, a practice that no doubt affected the college's position on the pressing new issues of curricular reform. Dismissing the benefits of university affiliation and the value of the laboratory to medical research and practice, EMI pur-sued a course that widened the chasm dividing eclectic from modern medicine. While top-tier medical colleges were reaching out to incor-porate new curriculum emphasizing the laboratory sciences, EMI was only expanding its hours of clinical instruction. Most of the students' medical science came from lectures and demonstrations rather than from experimentation in the laboratory. To Locke's credit, he con-

Frederick John Locke, M.D. (1829–1903),
dean of EMI (1894–1903). Courtesy of
the Lloyd Library and Museum.

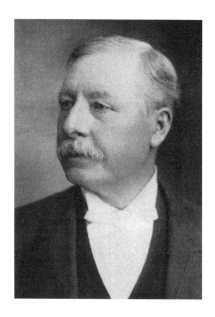

vinced the management to convert the first and second floors of the
college into a clinical amphitheater and free dispensary, and in 1901
he arranged for two hours of clinical instruction daily in the Cincinnati Hospital. Since EMI faculty were refused staff appointments
at the hospital, he negotiated with the Sisters of Charity to build
a three-story addition to Seton Hospital at 640 West Eighth Street
that included twelve patient rooms, an operating room, and clinical
amphitheater. There the faculty and students held forth on the principles of reform medicine.[36]

MASTODONS IN HARNESS

A student who entered EMI at the beginning of Locke's deanship
described the faculty as "abundantly endowed with the necessary
esteem of their own exalted ego," a description that applied to most
colleges—then and now. Each faculty member had his "peculiar, personal characteristics."[37] This depiction of the faculty could probably
have applied to just about any period in the school's history, with the
possible exception of the years between 1931 and 1939, when faculty

egos, as well as student antics, took a back seat to reorganization because of the dictates of the Association of American Medical Colleges, the Council on Medical Education of the American Medical Association, and increased standards set by state licensing boards.

The Locke years were decades of pride for EMI, capped with various successes, including the appointment of John K. Scudder to the Ohio State Board of Medical Registration and Examination (mixed board), incremental increases in the requirements for graduation, national reputations enjoyed by several of the faculty, renovations to the college's classrooms, increased numbers of applications, and the continued publication of textbooks by the faculty.[38]

Those eclectic works authored by the college's faculty included Andrew Jackson Howe's *The Diagnosis and Treatment of Dislocations and Fractures* (1870), *Diseases of the Eye* (1874), and *The Art and Science of Surgery* (1876); John A. Jeancon's *Anatomical Atlas* (1880) and *Pathological Atlas* (1882); John King's *The American Eclectic Obstetrics* (1855, 1876), *Woman, Her Diseases and Their Treatment* (1858), *The American Eclectic Dispensatory* (1861–62, 1870), *The Diagnosis and Treatment of Chronic Diseases* (1866), and *Urological Dictionary* (1878); John Uri Lloyd's *Chemistry of Medicines* (1881); and John M. Scudder's *A Practical Treatise on Diseases of Women* (1857), *Materia Medica and Therapeutics* (1858–59), *The Eclectic Practice of Medicine* (1863), *The Eclectic Practice of Medicine for Families* (1866), *The Principles of Medicine* (1867), *On the Use of Inhalations* (1867), *The Eclectic Practice of Medicine in Diseases of Children* (1869), *On the Reproductive Organs and the Venereal* (1874), *Specific Medication and Specific Medicines* (1870), and *Specific Diagnosis* (1874).

The early 1900s were transition years for the college faculty. Still teaching at EMC were the old war-horses, beloved by students, skeptical of the newer laboratory-based sciences, and anxious to finish their careers in their favorite chair. Along with these stalwarts were a handful of young, well-educated physicians (some with postgraduate experience) less concerned with the differences that distinguished eclectic from allopathic medicine than they were to obtain recognition from the Association of American Medical Colleges, the AMA's Council on Medical Education, and discipline-based professional organizations. For these faculty, peer recognition became a sine qua non for their continued allegiance to the college. Between these two extremes were the majority of the teaching and clinical faculty, who recognized that national standards were changing and who participated as reluctant players in medical innovation. Fearful of the impact that new challenges would have on the college and on their own personal lives, they tended to move slowly, hoping the change would be moderate, if not benign.

Foremost among the faculty were the so-called "Seven" who served as the mainstay of the college from the 1870s until the First World War: John M. Scudder, John King, Andrew Jackson Howe, Edwin Freeman, Frederick John Locke, John Allord Jeancon, and John Uri Lloyd.

Professor of surgery, Edwin Freeman (1834–1904), whose offices were at 51 West Seventh Street, taught medicine for nearly half a century. Knowledgeable of Thomsonism and botanic medicine in general, he resolved to enter EMI where his brother Zoheth was a professor. He matriculated in the winter of 1854–55 and graduated in 1856, becoming a close friend of John Milton Scudder, a fellow student. Freeman set up a successful practice in Cincinnati and in 1857 became demonstrator of anatomy at his alma mater. When the Civil War broke out, he was appointed assistant surgeon in the U.S. Volunteers and assigned to the Army of the Potomac, where he saw duty at the Battle of Fredericksburg and later campaigns in Virginia and central Kentucky. After the war, he moved to New York City as professor of anatomy in the Eclectic Medical College but returned in 1871 to his alma mater where he taught until 1899, assisted in later years by his son, E. R. Freeman. Known affectionately as the "noble old warhorse," he was always ready to do his share and was singularly unflappable when it came to student pranks. The constant din of student noise seemed not to affect him in the least. Four days each week, he gave lectures to the second- and third-year students on the most approved methods of operating. His lectures were illustrated by charts, models, and operations on cadavers. Sympathetic to his age and infirmities, students seldom annoyed this "aged veteran in the cause" and were well aware that only his feeble body hampered his abilities as a teacher.[39]

Professor John A. Jeancon (1831–1903) of 144 York Street in Newport, Kentucky, was a tall and powerfully built man who walked with the aid of a cane. Born in France, he went to school in Germany and Italy where he studied the classics before entering Middlesex Hospital Medical School in London and qualifying for practice in 1854.

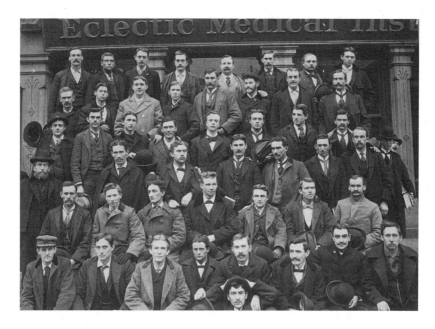

Class picture, 1890s. Professor Edwin Freeman (1834–1904) is at the far left in the third row. Courtesy of the Lloyd Library and Museum.

On coming to America, he engaged in practice until commissioned in 1861 as assistant surgeon in the Indiana Volunteers. Following an injury, the army sent him to Evansville, Indiana, where he served as the acting superintendent of several general hospitals. When Surgeon General William A. Hammond struck mercury and tartar emetic from the army supply table, Jeancon was included among the physicians appointed to investigate the indiscriminate usage of the two drugs. In 1865, he resumed private practice until 1874, when he was appointed to the chair of physiology and chemistry at EMI. In 1878, he took the chair of physiology, and then in 1891 that of pathology and pathological anatomy; finally, in 1898, he became clinical instructor in venereal diseases and diseases of the chest.

A "gentleman of great learning," Jeancon was nonetheless a "decided failure" as a disciplinarian in the three lectures he gave each week to the second- and third-year students. The mischief-loving students looked forward to his class "with true delight," stopping him midway during a lecture on pathology with a question "for the sake of information." With his "French blood boiling within him," recalled a graduate, Jeancon did not hesitate "to call the whole bunch . . . a set of d—— asses, or to hurl some other similarly effective epithet at them; or, taking his cane by the end furthest from the handle, threaten to clean out the entire outfit with it."[40]

By far the most famous of the school's faculty was professor of chemistry and pharmacy John Uri Lloyd (1849–1936), of Court and Plum Streets in Cincinnati, a teacher small in stature, faultlessly dressed, and always sporting a small nosegay in the left lapel of his coat. Without fanfare, he entered the classroom and, "with a quick, quiet, elastic step," mounted the platform and took control. Concerned with the welfare of the college in all its details, he would glance over the daily bulletin, looking for special announcements, and then turn to the blackboard for the outline of the day's lesson that had been prepared by his assistant, Harvey W. Felter. Approaching the table at the edge of the platform, he would check the instruments that Felter had set up for demonstration, inspecting closely to make sure that everything was in order. When satisfied that all was right, he rapped lightly on the table with his knuckles and began his lecture with a stereotypical, "Ladies and Gentlemen, . . ."[41]

John Uri recalled that when he first entered the institute in 1878, he had been warned by Scudder that the students, none of whom were "lambs," intended to take him "by the heels and shoulders and butt [him] against the wall, as they had done some other people." Resolving not to become their foil, he entered the classroom and, looking directly at the point of disturbance, pointed his finger and said, "Listen . . . I am here to teach you chemistry and you are here to learn chemistry. Either you will listen to me this hour through, in quiet, or I shall leave the room, never again to come back. You must make your choice now."[42] Lloyd gave three lectures per week to first- and second-year students. The course centered on medical chemistry, which he illustrated with experiments, giving special attention to chemical examination of urine, and to poisons and their antidotes.[43]

Lloyd's most unusual idiosyncracy was his refusal to permit students to take notes during lectures. Accordingly, pencils and notebooks were forbidden. He demanded courteous attention. "I shall give it to you," he said, and "you must give it to me." He warned that any student who threw a paper ball across the room would be reported to the board of trustees and expelled for insubordination. "Either [the culprit] will leave the college or the class will get no further instruction

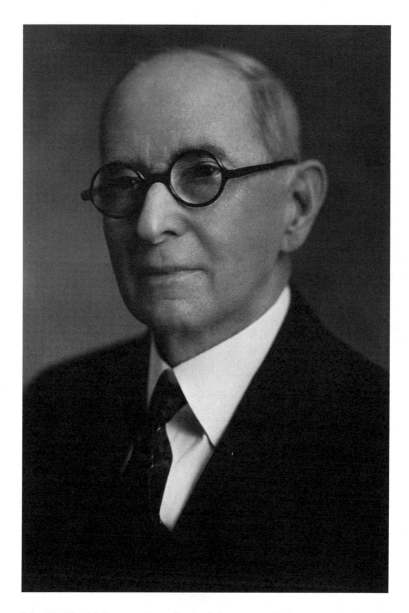

John Uri Lloyd (1849–1936), professor of chemistry and pharmacy, member and chairman of EMI's board of trustees, and principal benefactor along with brothers Curtis Gates Lloyd and Nelson Ashley Lloyd. Courtesy of the Lloyd Library and Museum.

from me." He promised to hear any student provided that he raised his hand for permission to speak. Anything else, even a whisper, was considered unacceptable behavior. Lloyd prohibited whistling during a lecture, promising to report any such incident to the board of trustees. Close attention was a prerequisite, for he followed each lecture with a quiz. "I had only to stop in the middle of a sentence," he once remarked, "and look at the inattentive party to make him wish he could sink through the floor."[44]

When Rolla L. Thomas first heard John Uri lecture in 1894, he knew at once that the college had a teacher of "unusual ability." Not only did Lloyd possess the knowledge of the subject matter, but he had the ability to impart that knowledge, as well as the gift of patience to get the principles of chemistry and pharmacy into "the most stupid pupils." Lloyd also was a good disciplinarian who possessed a gentleness and refinement that commanded both respect and attention. At any time, recalled Thomas, "you could have heard a pin drop when he was giving his lectures."[45]

Students recognized that "they were sitting at the feet of a master— one towering head and shoulders above his fellows in the realms of chemistry and pharmacy." While there was nothing fearful in his demeanor, students paid him respectful attention and Lloyd used only the force of reason, seldom changing the inflection of his voice to make a particular point. Only once did students act up in his class. On that occasion, Lloyd waited until the noise subsided and then informed the class that he would not attempt to match his voice against their combined efforts; whereupon he directed Felter to take over the class by quizzing them for the remainder of the hour. Without showing anger, he took his hat and left the room.[46]

Early in his professional career, John Uri became friends with John King and John M. Scudder, and, as this friendship matured, Lloyd identified with the cause of eclecticism and devoted his wholesale drug firm Lloyd Brothers (1885) and later Lloyd Brothers, Pharmacists, Inc. (1924) to the manufacture of specific medicines. From 1878 to 1907, John Uri held the chair of chemistry and pharmacy at the institute. In 1883, the Cincinnati College of Pharmacy appointed him to a similar position, which he resigned in 1887. That same year he was elected president of the American Pharmaceutical Association, a compliment to both Lloyd and to eclecticism. Among his many honors, Lloyd was appointed special member of the United States Pharmacopoeial

Commission and received three Ebert prizes (1882, 1891, 1916) for his work in pharmacy. In 1920, the American Pharmaceutical Association also awarded him their highest honor, the Remington Medal, for lifetime achievement.

The company that Lloyd owned in partnership with his two brothers sold American botanicals and was dedicated to replacing foreign drugs with American-made medicines.[47] Lloyd took exception to the older botanic belief that nature provided medicines for every ailment. "I feel that man is just one incident in passing," Lloyd wrote, "and that he must learn to utilize what may be about him. Far from having nature serve these things to his delectation, he must often make his discovery of them in the face of the resistance of nature herself."[48]

The breadth of Lloyd's scholarly interests made his lectures far different from the ordinary chemistry course taught in medical schools. His achievements ranged from basic research in colloidal chemistry, plant pharmacy, phytochemistry, drug extraction, and alkaloids to scientific articles in medical journals; and from the invention of the cold still (1904) for the distillation of plant medicines to authorship in 1895 of a science fiction romance, *Etidorhpa: Or, the End of the Earth* (from Aphrodite spelled backward), a historical story of Kentucky folklore in black dialect called *Stringtown on the Pike* (1900), and numerous other novels and scientific treatises and the founding of the Lloyd Pharmaceutical Library in Cincinnati. A man of great inquisitiveness, he instilled in students an awe of pharmacy, chemistry, and of the sciences in general, and the realization that the full measure of a medical student lay in his appreciation of the arts and humanities. Lloyd's fiction, while certainly not considered great literature, was popular in its day and garnered the approbation of some of the era's literary elite, including James Lane Allen and James Whitcomb Riley. His *Etidorhpa* (1895) remains in print to the present day, a favorite of New Age occultists.[49]

One of the first texts to come to the attention of students was Lloyd's *Chemistry of Medicine* (1881), his first book-length treatise and one of the earliest American textbooks on the subject. It remained the mainstay of the college's required texts for more than thirty years, going through eight editions. Other books included *Drugs and Medicines of North America* (1884), which he co-authored with his brother C. G. Lloyd; *King's Dispensatory* (1885), with John King; and *History of the Vegetable Drugs of the Pharmacopoeia of the United States* (1911,

1920). With these publications, John Uri became a preeminent authority on American plant remedies.[50]

John Uri was a valued contributor to the *Eclectic Medical Journal*, publishing his first article in the journal in 1870 on the simple and compound syrups of stillingia. After that, he wrote at least one article in every issue for a period of fifty-two years. In all, he wrote 644 articles for the journal. He contributed to every major pharmaceutical journal in the United States and many foreign journals as well. An index of his publications lists more than 3,500 in over fifty-two years. This includes 144 editorials for the *Eclectic Medical Gleaner* (1904–12), 104 articles on topics in lay journals, and 129 essays on various topics in the proceedings of the Cincinnati Literary Club during the twenty-five years he was a member.[51]

Two longtime friends of John Uri were merchant A. J. Conroy and attorney Frank Shaffer. The three met daily for luncheon in the Cincinnati Club, where they were known as the "Three Cronies." They were also members of the Old Tuesday Club that met in Hoffmann's winehouse at Race Street and Washington Park. The club included William Howard Taft, Elliott Pendleton, Albert Bettinger, and Judges Howard Hollister, John Weld Peck, and Alfred K. Nippert.[52]

Lloyd died in 1936, a week before his eighty-seventh birthday. Until his death, he remained an active member of the Cincinnati Academy of Eclectic Medicine, the Ohio State Eclectic Medical Association, the National Eclectic Medical Association, and the Alumnal Association of the college. His passing was felt deeply by the faculty, trustees, students, and alumni of the college. A self-made, self-disciplined man, he remained faithful throughout his life to the teachings of reform medicine. He had wide and diverse personal friendships with such luminaries as New York pharmacist Charles Rice (1841–1901); editor, author, and modernizer of pharmacy education Edward Kremers (1865–1941); and dean of the Philadelphia College of Pharmacy and a leader of the American Pharmaceutical Association, Joseph P. Remington (1847–1918). He also enjoyed fishing excursions with Grover Cleveland and visits from European scientists like German colloid chemist Wolfgang Ostwald and Swiss pharmacognosist Friedrich August Flückiger. Historian Glenn Sonnedecker described Lloyd as "one of the greatest and most versatile pharmacists that America has had." This depiction, while richly deserved, stands in sharp contrast to the sectarian community he championed.[53]

NEW BLOOD

Along with the "Seven" who led the school through its renaissance years were a number of new colleagues who contributed materially to the college's growth in the years before and after the First World War. Among them was professor of clinical surgery and operative gynecology Linus E. Russell (1849–1917), whose offices were located at "The Groton" in Cincinnati. Russell was a handsome man, tall, well built, with "a roguish glint in his eye." Born in Burton, Ohio, he spent his early life on a farm near where the Cuyahoga River empties into Lake Erie. At sixteen he entered Hiram College where he attended the lectures of James A. Garfield. In 1870, while teaching school in Mecca, Ohio, he began the study of medicine and in 1871 entered EMI, graduating a year later. Author of numerous papers on surgery and medical jurisprudence, and principal surgeon at Seton Hospital in Cincinnati, he accepted a chair at EMI in 1895. He brought to each weekly lecture and clinic an assortment of the latest instruments to demonstrate to students. He was an imposing personality, notwithstanding his disregard for "linguistics or philological niceties."[54]

By contrast, contempt for minor surgery was evident in the "high carnival" manner with which students treated professor Edgar T. Behymer (1855–1933), chair of general and clinical surgery. A graduate of EMI in 1881, he began practicing in Batavia, Ohio, before returning to teach at the college. Behymer was a young, stern German and his attempts to curb the students' "hell-bent inclinations" simply made matters worse; they indulged in all sorts of pranks at his expense. Seniors carried out most of the intrigues, although they found willing participants among their "mischievous younger brethren." Once, just before class, several pranksters adorned an old skeleton suspended from the ceiling of one of the large classrooms. They placed a stetson on its head, a cigar between its teeth, an umbrella between its ribs, and left it dangling so that Behymer could not help but bump into it upon entering the lecture room. When that occurred, he snapped at the students: "I'll goose-egg every one of you; remember I hold this book [the roll book]." Had Behymer not reacted so predictably, the students might have left him alone. He soon left the college, resigning in 1897 to move into general practice.[55]

Clinical professor of didactic surgery William E. Bloyer (1853–1923), whose offices were located at "The Lancaster" on 22 West Seventh

Street, graduated from EMI in 1879. An imposing man, he tipped the scales at three hundred pounds. His presence inspired awe in the average medical student, many of whom "needed just such a reminder of the proper relationship between teacher and pupil." However, Bloyer did not need his imposing figure to impress upon students that they give their undivided attention to his lectures on anatomy. Having gained a reputation for his knowledge of cerebral localization, he attracted the attention of both eclectics and regulars. A champion of eclectic principles, Bloyer once served as president of the National Eclectic Medical Association and of the Cincinnati Eclectic Medical Society.

Four days a week, beginning at 7:30 each morning, Bloyer greeted his class with a half-hour quiz on the previous day's lecture, followed by a new lecture. With a low, firm, and earnest voice, "he wielded a wonderful influence . . . reaching every fibre." On one occasion, a student tried to demonstrate that the hour's lecture was nearly over by opening and closing his watch case. "Snap your tin-case all you like, you shallow-pated cuss," he said. "I don't stop till I am through." He then proceeded to give a fifteen-minute sermon, concluding with the remark: "Some of you come here, sent perhaps by wealthy parents who are anxious that you should obtain a valuable education; lazy and trifling yourselves, you must even annoy those who come here to learn. I tell you, that some of you will see the time when you may wish you could drop through a knot-hole in the floor, some day when you are confronted by intelligent, learned men, and in need of the very knowledge you fail to receive here, because of just such inattention." Students appreciated Bloyer because he was reasonable in his demands, hated dishonesty, and had little patience for the student who tried to "ride a pony" through his particular branch of studies.[56]

Robert C. Wintermute (1861–1906), whose offices were situated at 129 West Seventh Street, was clinical professor of obstetrics, gynecology, and pediatrics. He received his literary education at Union College before graduating from EMI in 1881. He lectured five times each week to second- and third-year students and held a clinic each week where students familiarized themselves with various instruments and prescribed remedies. A tall and stately man, he impressed upon students that what he did not know about obstetrics and gynecology was probably not worth learning. Every lecture included his dexterous manipulation of a mannequin on the table before him. With it, he demonstrated the varying problems that confronted the accoucheur. Always looking over his spectacles, he surveyed the class for the omnipresent mischief maker; at the proper moment, he would take a seat on a high stool next to the mannequin while the troublesome student, "having drawn his card of chance at the Wintermute lottery," would be given a problem presentation in birth. "With beads of perspiration standing out from every pore," the hapless student would try to demonstrate his knowledge of obstetrics while the rest of the class eagerly watched. Any "hisses or signs of exultation from anyone" were promptly and severely silenced.[57]

Professor of pathology and physiology Lyman Watkins (1854–1912) of Blanchester, Ohio, received his medical education at Starling Medical College (regular) in Columbus, Ohio, and then converted to eclecticism. He would enter the lecture room with "firm, measured steps" and, casting his glance over the assembled class, pick out an "obdurate colt" or an "unsuspecting enemy" who he would proceed to "paralyze" with questions. Though tough, he was a fair teacher with a distaste for cocky students "brimming full and running over with smartness." Watkins knew all the students by name, and anyone who attempted to slip out unnoticed through the back door before the lecture concluded would receive a rude awakening. "That was Mr. so-and-so," he would say, then open his roll book and proceed to place "a beautiful goose-egg" opposite the student's name. Assisted by G. W. Brown, he conducted two general medical clinics each week where students learned diagnosis and eclectic treatment based on the doctrines of specific medication.[58]

Professor of medical jurisprudence William L. Dickson (1856–1895), whose offices were at 702 Union Trust Building, graduated from Yale College in 1878 and returned to his hometown of Cincinnati where he read law and was admitted to the bar in 1881. In 1890, he was appointed lecturer in medical jurisprudence and was reputed to have a tongue "like a two-edged sword." Those who wished to ask a question were required to write it out and send it forward to the podium. His responses ranged from sarcastic and severe, to scathing, moral, and "mind your own business." Since he dealt with the legal issues of medicine, he escaped much of the roasting received by his medical colleagues. Often he would say to the students: "You doctors are used to dealing with only children, sick and dying people who can offer no resistance; you are used to having your own way; hence you can never stand opposition. If you were *lawyers*, you would find life's battle a little different."[59]

Students considered William Byrd Scudder (1869–1905), professor of ophthalmology and otology, whose office was located in the Neave Building, one of the school's finest instructors. Born in Avondale, Ohio, in 1869, he attended Cincinnati University for two years before transferring to EMI where he graduated in 1890. He attended sessions on ophthalmology and otology at the New York Post-Graduate Medical School and Hospital and later studied at Moorfield's Ophthalmic Hospital in London and at the Allegemeine Clinic in Vienna, Austria. A natural teacher, Scudder spoke to the subject and not just about it. He conducted one lecture each week to second- and third-year students and one clinic each week giving special attention to the techniques of specific medication. Clear in his diction, he was always able to elucidate any point he wished to make and avoid bombast. Closest in age to the students, he captured their attention with lectures that were "short, clear and pithy," followed by the inevitable quizzes that were practical and directly to the point. A teacher blessed with patience, he lacked this quality only when dealing with dunces. On those occasions, he would pull out his pencil and begin drawing Os in his grade book.[60]

Also among the faculty was Professor William N. Mundy (1860–1946) of Forest, Ohio. A small man, but "large in mind," he was a keen observer, distant from students, impatient, and a proverbial "bundle of nerves." Born in New Jersey in 1860, he received his education in the public schools of New York City and entered New York College in 1874. After moving to Ohio, he began the study of medicine and graduated from EMI in 1883 and then took additional study at the New York Post-Graduate Medical School and Hospital. The facts that he laid before students may have been clear in his own mind, but most found him difficult to understand. Those few students who followed his "rapid-firing methods" benefited from his didactic skills; unfortunately, few were capable of realizing this. Mundy lasted only a short time, resigning in 1897, whereupon he returned to Forest and set up a highly successful practice.[61]

Professor Bishop McMillen (1856–1911), an expert alienist and neurologist from Columbus, Ohio, taught mental and nervous diseases and delivered twelve lectures each session. A graduate of EMI in 1881, he practiced medicine for seven years before securing an appointment at the Columbus State Hospital for the Insane—the first eclectic physician in Ohio to obtain a position in a state asylum. In 1894, he became associated with Shephard's Sanitarium and in that same year was appointed to the EMI faculty. Few chairs were considered more important in the late nineteenth century, and students of eclectic practice seemed especially interested in the effects of "the strenuous life" on American workers. As a neurologist with an extensive private practice in sanitaria, McMillen brought to the classroom a broad array of case histories. His class "was eagerly anticipated, and it never failed to be a period of real satisfaction to the zealous student."[62]

After teaching for several years in the Ohio public schools, John R. Spencer (1854–1924) began the study of medicine and graduated from EMI in 1881. Having established a successful practice at 952 West Eighth Street, he was invited back to his alma mater to teach electrotherapeutics, hygiene, and physical diagnosis to second- and third-year students. A dedicated eclectic, he served as president of the local and national eclectic medical associations. Spencer seemed ill suited to his discipline, since students judged him neither "surcharged with magnetism nor yet a walking electric dynamo." His lectures were "dry and uninteresting," and, not surprisingly, he was an easy target for the boisterously inclined who, by the end of the day, were ready for merriment. With the "patience of Job," he would talk about his various cases, but student antics meant that little was actually learned in the class. At exam time, however, students passed with the same difficulty that the proverbial Dutchman got into heaven—"mit a damned dight schqueeze."[63]

Another popular teacher was Harvey Wickes Felter (1865–1933), who came from Albany County, New York, where he obtained a teacher's certificate and divided his time between farming and teaching. In 1883, he studied medicine under the tutelage of an old-school physician in New York but soon adopted the eclectic system against the advice of friends. He graduated from EMI in 1888 and then located in Troy, New York, for a year before returning to Cincinnati where he was first appointed demonstrator of anatomy, quizmaster in chemistry, as well as assistant to John Uri in pharmacy. Eventually, he became professor of chemistry and toxicology and professor of materia medica and therapeutics. His office was located at 1733 Chase Street, Northside.

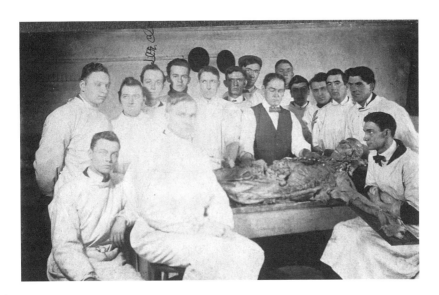

Students with a cadaver, ca. 1890. Courtesy of the Lloyd Library and Museum.

Among his many duties, Felter became the unofficial historian of the college and contributed regularly to the *Eclectic Medical Journal.* Though physically very different from Lloyd, the young Felter had so absorbed the expressions and mode of thinking of his mentor that he seemed to students to exude most of the qualities and tendencies of Lloyd. "The manner of expression, extreme accuracy, pronunciation, enunciation and all else tending to clearly impress upon the students the exact information sought" were characteristics of both men. Known to be an "ideal quizmaster," Felter never used his authority to trick students with an unfair question. He held two recitations and quizzes each week for first- and second-year students.[64]

The most repulsive aspect of medical studies was dissection. Yet, as a demonstrator of anatomy, Felter was appreciated by most EMI students. Always willing to guide "the boys" through this "nasty, horrible work," he never failed to explain every point as fully as possible. At the end of each exercise, students gathered around him as he used a hand punch to perforate the number in the margin of their dissecting card that corresponded to the question they answered correctly.[65]

The quietest spot in the college was the laboratory of Professor George W. Brown (1869–1908), demonstrator of histology and pathology and, later, bacteriology. From Newport, Kentucky, he studied medicine under Professor Frederick J. Locke before attending EMI and graduating in 1890. After three months of additional study at the New York Post-Graduate Medical School and Hospital, he returned to Newport where he maintained a practice at 239 East Fifth Street. In 1895, he succeeded Watkins as demonstrator of the microscopical laboratory. Here students spent hours peering into their individual microscopes "instead of making googoo eyes at the lady students." Brown instructed them in the use of the microscope, the mounting of specimens, and the normal and abnormal histological appearances of body tissues. The class itself was divided into sections of sixteen to ensure adequate space in the laboratory. Colleagues sometimes begrudged Brown his quiet laboratory since too many of them had to face the more boisterous side of students. Brown's specimens were much prized and, surprisingly, his class was always a picture of decorum. Seldom did he suffer from student pranks. No doubt the cost of equipment and the potential for breakage served as a clear and obvious deterrent.[66]

Scudder Brothers

In 1906, the Scudder brothers reduced the capital stock in their corporation from twenty dollars a share to six dollars, returning fourteen dollars into the treasury of the corporation. In taking this action, they transferred the building on Plum Street to the Scudder Brothers Corporation in return for each brother handing over 175 shares each of the capital stock. This left John K. Scudder with 225 shares and Paul R. Scudder with 75 shares. For all practical purposes, "John K" *was* the institute, making nearly all administrative decisions—from admissions and hiring faculty to setting salaries and tuition.[67]

At a special meeting of the stockholders on December 19, 1908, the brothers surrendered all of the outstanding shares of capital stock in order to permit the college to continue its existence as a not-for-profit within the provisions of Ohio law. With the two remaining stockholders (John K. and Paul R. Scudder) present at the meeting, one brother offered a resolution, the other seconded, and the two

John King Scudder, M.D. (1865–1930),
secretary, treasurer, and operating officer
of Eclectic Medical Institute and College
(1888–1929). Courtesy of the Lloyd
Library and Museum.

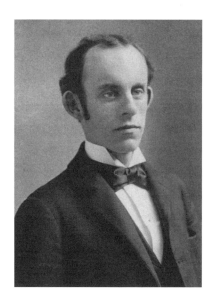

voted that "we and each of us do hereby surrender to the Eclectic
Medical Institute . . . the shares of stock now owned by us."[68]

Following the change to a not-for-profit corporation, John K. Scudder remained as secretary and treasurer of the college at a salary of six
hundred dollars a year. Born in Cincinnati, he was educated in the
Avondale public schools and received his A.B. from Cincinnati University in 1882 and his medical degree from EMI in 1888. That same
year, he became secretary to the faculty and the board of trustees
of the college. In addition, Professor "John K" served as an instructor
in Latin and prescription writing from 1894 to 1897 and director of
the laboratories and clinics and took over duties as managing editor of
the *Eclectic Medical Journal* following the death of his father. Later, he
became director of the laboratories and clinics. Young Scudder was a
lucid writer whose editorials were greatly prized by students. "His large
forehead, outstanding ears, keen eyes, prominent nose, closed lips and
bright intellect" were traits handed down from his father.[69]

But the years that Scudder managed the college also represented a
watershed in the history of the school, as it was abundantly clear to
the faculty and its board of trustees that medical education was changing. In the aftermath of licensing criteria established by the Illinois

Board of Health in 1877, and with the reactivation of the Association of American Medical Colleges in 1890 and the muscles flexed by the Council on Medical Education of the American Medical Association, medical schools began upgrading their admission standards and curriculum. These changes were already evident in top-tier schools, and numerous second- and third-tier schools were feeling the implications of these changes on their own institutions.

In the year 1909–10, tuition receipts for EMC amounted to $7,012.46, with instructional costs of $2,446.90. This did not include professor fees of $2,645, an annual salary of $600 for John K. Scudder, office expenses of $559, and insurance of $576. Nonetheless, these figures represented a typical year, leaving little in the budget to finance research, support scholarships, or purchase needed laboratory equipment. At the end of four years (1908–12), total tuition receipts for the college amounted to $29,737.53, with expenses for the four years at $29,176.75, leaving a balance of $560.78 for the endowment fund.[70] Salaries for the faculty were never large. In 1912, Rolla L. Thomas received $140 for his lectures on the practice of medicine and $140 for his service as dean. At the low end of the scale, William L. Dickson received an annual stipend of $25 for his lectures on medical jurisprudence; W. E. Postle received $52.50 for his course on mental and nervous diseases; A. J. Nunnamaker received $75 as demonstrator in anatomy; and E. B. Shewman received $210 for his course on anatomy and surgery. The only full-time instructor in 1912 was F. B. Grosvenor, who received $675 for teaching histology, pathology, and bacteriology.[71]

The essentials of scientific medicine consisted of basic science faculty, research laboratories and assistants, increased clinical hours, and alternative sources of funding. For any number of second- and third-tier proprietary and university-affiliated medical schools, however, staffing consisted of adjunct faculty taking time out of their busy practices to prepare the next generation of practitioners. Research was certainly permissive—even laudatory—in these schools and departments but not essential to their educational missions. These were community-based schools that produced trained practitioners, not specialists. Few of these schools shared Abraham Flexner's vision of medicine as research oriented; nor did they appreciate the relationship that Flexner and other admirers of German university education had drawn between experimental science and medical questions. It was not that they distrusted the laboratory sciences; rather, they believed that medical education was best learned in the examining room of the clinic, dispensary, or family doctor. American medicine (both regular and sectarian) moved ever so slowly from the Paris clinical model, with its focus on bedside observation, to the German model of experimental laboratory investigation. By the time of Flexner's examination of medical education in the United States and Canada, the foundation for a German-based educational system was largely in place in American universities.

For the eclectics, this transition never materialized. Despite their rhetoric, the American school of reform medicine had not even managed to fulfill the spirit of the Paris clinical model. Unable to establish strong staff and teaching relationships in the large urban hospitals, they were forced to settle for minor hospitals, dispensaries, and private practices as the source of their clinical education. Because of these limitations, eclectic medicine remained impoverished by the standards of both the Paris and German educational models.

CHAPTER THREE

Academics

Dᴜʀɪɴɢ ᴛʜᴇ ᴘᴇʀɪᴏᴅ that Scudder, King, and Howe were reestab-
lishing the principles of eclecticism following the debacle over
concentrated medicines, the top tier of American medical schools
began the task of adjusting to the impact of academic medicine. In
1859, the medical department of Lind University in Chicago reformed
its medical program by instituting a sequential curriculum as an alternative to the standard two four-month terms of lectures, with the second identical to the first. The college also required the presence of
a sound preliminary education. This initial effort proved short lived
since most medical departments concluded that all must reform, or
none. There were simply too many options available to the aspiring
doctor for a few schools to break from standard practices.[1]

In 1871, President Charles W. Eliot (1834–1926) of Harvard, trained
as a chemist and a longtime admirer of German education, renewed
the reform effort by insisting that the medical school at Harvard become a more integral part of the university by placing faculty on regular salaries, introducing a graded curriculum, replacing the school's
two-year program with a three-year extended teaching term, and requiring higher admission standards. Other reforms followed, pushed
by forward-thinking administrators and individual faculty who sought
to professionalize their respective disciplines and specializations. Fran-
cis Delafield and William H. Welch opened clinical laboratories in the
College of Physicians and Surgeons in New York and Bellevue Medical
College in 1878; and Yale and the University of Michigan followed in
1880 with laboratories in the experimental sciences. Provost William
Pepper of the University of Pennsylvania added another innovation
when he placed the University Hospital under the direct supervision of
the school's medical faculty. With this change, the hospital became an

integral part of the medical school and served the education of doctors as well as the needs of patients. Previously, students could only view operations from perches in an amphitheater; now, with the hospital under the exclusive control of the school's faculty, students profited from direct bedside teaching and residency in the medical and surgical clinics.

Added impetus came from scientific societies and groups of specialists such as the American Surgical Association (1880), the Association of American Physicians (1886), the American Physiological Society (1887), the American Association of Anatomists (1888), the Pediatric Society (1888), and the American Association of Pathologists and Bacteriologists (1900). These organizations formed from a need to further individual and group identity, advance pure and applied research, and encourage the exchange of scientific information. In doing so, they distanced their members from less credentialed practitioners.[2]

As university faculty and administrators caught the spirit of reform, they transformed academic medicine into a stronger pedagogy. By the 1890s, sixty or more of the 158 medical schools in existence were connected with universities. Admittedly, most of these medical schools still maintained their autonomy and controlled their finances, appointments, and standards for admission and graduation. Many of these same departments were located miles from the parent institution, with the only visible evidence of a connection, besides letterhead, being the annual appearance of the university president to confer degrees at commencement.[3]

Nevertheless, the nature of the relationship had begun to change, distinguished in large measure by the founding of Johns Hopkins Medical College in 1893 and the graduation of its first class of fifteen in 1897. Similar efforts flourished at Harvard, Yale, Columbia, Pennsylvania, Cornell, and Clark. Clearly, the increased costs of library collections, laboratory equipment, and salaried teachers in the fundamental branches of science justified the need for closer university ties. Medical faculty recognized that the "fundamentals," which constituted the first two years of the curriculum—physics, chemistry, anatomy, zoology, physiology, and bacteriology—were more efficiently and more thoroughly taught by university-trained faculty. Medicine had finally become an applied science demanding a firm foundation in the application of the principles, facts, and methods of the basic sciences.

As marginal as many of these university-based medical departments were by present-day standards, they were substantively better than proprietary colleges whose medical faculties attempted to teach the basic sciences in the context of short five- or six-month sessions on the assumption they were covering the knowledge essential for students' future needs. The old masters in these proprietary schools taught well what was then known, and, as Arthur Dean Bevan of Chicago noted in his remarks before the Aesculapian Club of Harvard in 1912, "their medical schools and their methods of teaching . . . were in keeping with the knowledge of their day."[4] But as medicine became an applied science, the older method of didactic lecture confined to a few fundamental branches no longer sufficed. Academic medicine demanded a more rigorous and disinterested viewpoint, laboratories equipped and organized like university laboratories devoted to nonmedical sciences, teachers scholarly in spirit and method, and students who approached the curriculum in an atmosphere that Abraham Flexner described as "freshened by the search for truth."[5]

But the benefits of university affiliation never became as pressing an issue for the faculty or the trustees of the eclectic college. Throughout the ninety-four-year history of the school, both were less interested in the investigative and research aspects of medicine than with the routine practices of diagnosis and treatment. The college depended on a cohort of former graduates who divided their time between the classroom and private practice. This, the trustees concluded, was more than sufficient. The function of a university-based medical school and the desire to extend the boundaries of knowledge by independent research remained ancillary to the preparation of good family practitioners.

ENTRANCE REQUIREMENTS

Through much of the nineteenth century, students who attended liberal arts colleges were clearly distinct from those who attended professional schools. The former had a broad array of subject prerequisites for admission, while applicants to professional schools could usually matriculate after just about any English secondary school course or enter directly from grammar school after a specified apprenticeship.[6] Beginning in 1870, certification began replacing the more traditional admission method of written and oral examinations before the president and faculty. Examination was waived for those students whose

high schools could certify their completion of a specified list of subject requirements. First initiated by the University of Michigan, this
opened the way for a more broadly based set of course requirements;
by the 1890s, certification had become a national phenomenon,
spreading as well to professional schools.[7]

Of the ninety-four regular medical schools in existence in 1890,
twenty-three had no requirements for matriculation; four required evidence of a fair or good English education; fifty-five required examination, or its equivalent, in the branches of an English education; and
the remainder required examination in the branches of an English
education and Latin (or occasionally another language). Of the ten
eclectic colleges, one required a common (grammar) school education
and nine required an examination in the English branches or, alternatively, a diploma from a high or normal school or academy, a teacher's
certificate, or the equivalent.[8]

Lack of uniformity in high schools meant that a high school degree
represented an uncertain standard at best. For most schools, the real
standard became "or the equivalent," which represented the minimum to which the quality of instruction conformed. Until the certification system brought greater uniformity to the curriculum, a young
man unable to attend high school could overcome that impediment
through a number of different avenues including examination by the
faculty of the institution to which he was seeking admission. For this
reason, and because so many colleges were lax in conducting entrance
examinations, states such as New York, Ohio, and Minnesota established an external examination under the auspices of an education department or a state board. In most states, these agencies were either
powerless or unwilling to antagonize schools by rigorously enforcing
the high school standard.[9]

In 1902, President Eliot of Harvard, discussing admission eligibility,
remarked: "I venture to say that any American university now in existence which does not require a college degree for admission to its
professional schools, will in twenty years find itself in an inferior position to those universities that do require it." His prediction proved
to be remarkably prescient; the criteria for admission was clearly being
raised.[10] In 1904, only four medical colleges (Johns Hopkins, Harvard, Western Reserve, and Rush) required education beyond high
school. By 1914, eighty-four colleges required one or more years of college work. Of the eighty-four, thirty-four required two or more years

MEDICAL STUDENT'S EXAMINATION.

Certificate of Preliminary Instruction.

Eclectic Medical Institute:

THIS CERTIFIES, That Mr. _____

(Give full name.)

of _____ a Student of _____

(Give residence.)   (Give name of School.)

has pursued successfully, to the extent indicated, the following studies that are not erased:

(To enter without conditions ten studies are sufficient. A student can enter on seven out of this list with three conditions to be made up before he can advance to the Sophomore medical class. The ten studies must include all in the column headed "required" and any two in the column of "electives.")

REQUIRED:	ELECTIVES:
Orthography.	General History, one year, or English History, or
Geography.	History of Greece and Rome.
English Grammar and Composition.	English Literature, one year.
History and Constitution of the United States.	Rhetoric, one year.
Arithmetic, including the Metric System and Men-	German, one year.
suration.	French, one year.
Algebra to Quadratics.	Latin (Cæsar, Virgil or Cicero), second years' work.
Latin (Grammar and Cæsar Book 1).	Physiology, one year.
Physics, elementary.	Chemistry, one year.
	Botany, one year.
(In addition to the above studies, two more must be certified to, the two to be chosen from the next column.)	Zoology, one year.
	Physical Geography, one year.
	Geometry, plane, one year.

Signed at _____

this _____ *day of* _____ *190_____*

_____

Principal, or Secretary, or Examiner.

NOT VALID WITHOUT SEAL OF THE SCHOOL, OF A COUNTY SUPERIN-TENDENT, OR A NOTARY PUBLIC.	(If the school has no seal, then the signature of the school officer must be witnessed by the Superintendent of Education with seal, or by a Notary Public with seal, on the form below.)

Executed in the presence of

_____ *190_____*   **DEC 1 0 1904**   *Notary Public or Supt. of Education.*

Hendricks printed 200 in Oct/1904

Medical student's certificate of preliminary instruction, 1904. Courtesy of the Lloyd Library and Museum.

for admission.[11] By the same year, thirteen state licensing and examining boards had adopted preliminary requirements beyond the four-year high school education.[12]

These statistics are deceptive, since there were measurable differences in the educational profiles of regular and sectarian students. While 23.5 percent of the graduates of regular medical schools began with A.B. or B.S. degrees by 1914, only 4.5 percent of the homeopathic graduates and 8.6 percent of the eclectic graduates had liberal arts degrees. During this same period, college terms lengthened. In 1901, one hundred colleges reported sessions of from twenty-three to twenty-eight weeks; only two colleges reported sessions shorter than twenty-nine weeks in 1914. Of the 101 colleges existing in 1904, 94.1 percent required from thirty-one to thirty-six weeks of actual work, compared with 30 percent in 1901.[13]

In the seventy-nine-year period from 1846 through 1924, the Eclectic Medical Institute graduated 4,212 students. The class of 1892, the first class scheduled for a three-year course of study, numbered fifty-two. The previous graduating class had seventy-five. After a two-year period during which the numbers of graduates declined, the enrollment again increased. The average size of the graduating class during these years was fifty-three, with a low of eight students in 1900, when the school moved to a four-year curriculum, and a high of one hundred and twenty-two in 1878. Seven states contributed the greatest number of students: Ohio, Indiana, New York, Pennsylvania, Illinois, Kentucky, and West Virginia.

Responding to the higher entrance requirements demanded by the Association of American Medical Colleges, the Eclectic Medical College provided specific policy in 1911 on admission credentials. These included a diploma from an approved college granting the degree of B.A. or B.S.; a certificate showing graduation from a high school of first grade and issued after four years of study; a teacher's permanent or life high school certificate; or a certificate of admission to the freshman class of an approved literary or scientific college. Disallowed were county, city, or village certificates to teach school; diplomas from high schools of less than first grade; diplomas or degrees from normal schools in which less than four years of work had been completed; or certifications that had not led to the conferring of a diploma or degree. Lacking an acceptable credential, prospective students could request certification by examination from the State Entrance Examiner. The examination, held once each year in Cincinnati, Columbus, Cleveland, and Toledo, tested students in English, Latin, history, mathematics, and science. A general average of 75 percent, with no grade below 60 percent, was the minimum for admittance to EMC. Theoretically this removed the temptation for the faculty or administrators of the institution to bend admission rules. However, the state examiner accepted several alternatives, including years taken in different institutions, provided they added to four, tutor-certificates testifying to the candidate's work, and examinations that covered less than the high school course.[14]

The actual admission standards listed in catalogs bore little resemblance to accepted practice in many if not most medical colleges. As noted earlier, the real standard was typically "or the equivalent." Complicating this situation, Ohio, Illinois, and many other states allowed preliminary educational requirements to be made up after admission. This meant that students could embark on their medical program while promising to fulfill deficiencies in their high school education at a convenient time afterward.[15] This was certainly true at EMI, where students entering in 1900 lacking the necessary admission credentials were required to take an examination before beginning the fall term. This consisted of an English composition of not less than two hundred words and testing in the areas of math, U.S. history, geography, elementary physics, and Latin. Students unable to pass tests in the latter two disciplines were permitted to study them during their first year of classes.[16]

By 1913, thirty-two medical schools required as a minimum for entrance two or more years of work in a college of liberal arts in addition to a four-year high school education; seven schools announced the adoption of the two-year collegiate requirement to take effect by 1914–15; twenty-one medical colleges announced the requirement of one year of college work in physics, chemistry, biology, and a modern foreign language; and another twenty-one hinted that, in addition to the standard four-year high school education, they would consider requiring a premedical college year devoted to courses in physics, chemistry, biology, and a modern language. Seventy-one medical colleges thus required at least one year of college work in physics, chemistry, biology, and a modern language. EMC was not among that group of colleges even though the list included one eclectic and two homeopathic schools.[17]

As late as 1914, EMC still admitted students with fifteen units from an accredited high school, as determined by the Ohio State Medical Board, with no obligatory premedical courses. In defense of the college's policy, John Uri Lloyd argued that all the university-based colleges of medicine could not, under the new standards, replace the annual loss of physicians. Nor were there sufficient applicants ready to take the proposed new curriculum. In his judgment, those who graduated under the approved plans of the AMA's Council on Medical Education would have advanced opportunities as specialists but would leave the nation's sparsely settled areas without sufficient health providers. Lloyd preferred a more "balanced" approach that would ensure the continued presence of the self-sacrificing general practitioner of olden times. Believing that medicine was being turned over to a mercenary cadre of specialists, he predicted that the vast majority of the nation's families would soon be left to the mercy of patent medicine advertisers. Lloyd did not intend to diminish the importance of university-educated physicians and specialists; rather, he advocated a system of medical education that would also ensure a future for the family physician.[18]

The college administration was fully aware of the need to bolster admission requirements and, in a letter to six hundred alumni, secretary John K. Scudder reported on these changes and urged them to recruit a cohort of students before Ohio increased entrance requirements beyond the present high school standard.[19] To assist prospective students in having this additional preparation, Scudder arranged with Earlham College in Richmond, Indiana, to provide these courses. Located seventy miles from Cincinnati, on the Chicago division of the Pennsylvania Railroad, Earlham offered a convenient location for this additional work. Room, board, and tuition at Earlham cost $270 per year.[20] Scudder sent letters out to some five hundred eclectic doctors practicing in Indiana informing them of EMC's arrangement with the Earlham faculty. Later, the college made similar arrangements with Defiance College in Defiance, Ohio; Bluffton College in Bluffton, Ohio; and Xavier College in Cincinnati.[21]

Not until 1920 were student matriculants at EMC required to show both a high school certificate and proof of premedical higher education. The Ohio Medical Students Entrance Certificate, which students obtained from the State Medical Board in Columbus for three dollars, required the student to have graduated from a first-grade high school and attended a "well recognized medical college" prior to 1914; or, show evidence of having taken one premedical college year or attended at least one year at another medical school between 1914 and 1917; or, show evidence of having taken two years of premedical college requirements, including physics, chemistry, biology, English, and one other modern language, equivalent to sixty college credit hours. Students applying to EMC presented their certificates and other credentials or credits at the time of matriculation.[22]

GRADUATION REQUIREMENTS

From 1845 to 1871, the minimum requirements for graduation at EMI included three years of reading with two sessions of lectures, or four years' practice and only one course of lectures. Between 1871 and 1878 the college revised its requirements, demanding three years of reading and two sessions of sixteen weeks with thirty-six lectures per week. During that time, and in subsequent years, faculty encouraged students in their preceptorships to read Joel Dorman Steele's *Fourteen Weeks in Physics* (1869), John Uri Lloyd's *The Chemistry of Medicines* (1881), William S. Kirkes's *Handbook of Physiology* (1860), John Bell's *Comparative Anatomy and Physiology* (1885), Henry Gray's *Anatomy, Descriptive and Surgical* (1859), Sanborn Tenney's *Natural History* (1866), and John M. Scudder's *Principles of Medicine* (1867), *Specific Medication and Specific Medicines* (1870) and *Specific Diagnosis* (1874). During this same period, the regular session commenced in October and the spring session in February, one week after the close of the winter session. Matriculation, tuition, and a demonstrator's ticket cost seventy dollars; the graduation fee was twenty-five dollars, and board was available for about four to five dollars per week. Alternatively, students could purchase a "certificate of scholarship" for $125, entitling them to attend as many courses of lectures as they wished prior to graduation.[23] In an effort to establish a place among competing schools in the 1870s, EMI explained to prospective students that, unlike other medical colleges, it had not chosen to increase the numbers of students by "advertising a large corps of professors." Instead, EMI provided "one capable teacher in each department [and] we regard [this] as much better than two or three."[24]

When it became clear that students were matriculating without the benefit of preceptorships, a factor common to both regular and sectarian schools in the second half of the nineteenth century, the college decided to provide for the student's entire medical education. For a small additional cost, the college offered students the option of attending a two-year course of study (four sessions of lectures) while simultaneously working in a local physician's office. This, the faculty reasoned, was better preparation for practice than the ordinary three years of reading and two sessions of lectures, or, one course of lectures and four years of practice.[25] By the 1880s, however, the faculty reported that full-time enrollment without office instruction had produced many of the college's more successful physicians. With that admission, the college made no further efforts to continue with the optional office instruction.[26]

After the spring and winter sessions of 1880–81, the faculty announced that three courses of lectures were required for graduation; those who came with practical experience could attend only two sessions. The regular session commenced in September and continued for twenty weeks, with the spring session starting in late January and closing in early June. This schedule provided for nineteen weeks of lectures (thirty-six lectures each week and an additional twelve hours of hospital experience) and one week for examinations.[27] Fees increased another five dollars per session; alternatively, students could purchase a three-year course of tickets for $150. Graduates from other medical colleges were admitted to lectures on half fees while graduates of EMI were admitted free. Women were admitted on the same terms as men beginning in 1874, but decorum required that they be provided their own private entrance and reception room.[28]

By 1890, two new laboratories were added in chemistry and histology, and, for the first time, the college advertised two need-based scholarships awarded on the basis of competitive examinations. The faculty also notified students that, following the 1893–94 session, the requirements for graduation would increase once again. Although there would be no change in the length of the session or in fees, students were required to read medicine for four years, including attendance in three annual courses of lectures of not less than six months each, the last of which had to be at the institute. These curricular revisions, required by changes in state licensing laws and pressures from the Association of American Medical Colleges and the Council on Medical Education, came as an unwelcome intrusion in the students' already busy schedules. A year later, however, the college again raised its requirements, lengthening the sessions from six months to eight.[29]

In its 1901 bulletin, EMI explained that entrance requirements were in accord with those of the Association of American Medical Colleges, the Homeopathic College Association, and the National Confederation of Eclectic Medical Colleges. The bulletin detailed the current state laws for medical licensing, announced a new schedule of fees as well as room and board information, explained library privileges, and identified hospital and clinical facilities. The bulletin also devoted considerable attention to the clinical instruction available daily in the Cincinnati Hospital, the surgical operations performed in the college amphitheater, the work conducted at the dispensary at 6735 Kenyon Avenue, and the arrangements made with the Sisters of Charity for the exclusive use of Seton Hospital at 640 West Eighth and Cutter.[30]

The schedule of hours for students in the 1900–1901 session listed the following:[31]

FIRST YEAR HOURS

Hygiene	26	Chemical Laboratory	39
Anatomy	104	Dissections	78
Chemistry	52	Latin	26
Physiology	52	Physics	26
Materia Medica	104	Total	507

SECOND YEAR HOURS

Dissection	39	Principles of Medicine	26
Anatomy	104	Hygiene	26
Physiology	52	Physical Diagnosis	26
Chemistry	52	Electro-Therapeutics	26
Materia Medica	104	Hospital Clinics	312
		Total	767

THIRD YEAR HOURS

Electro-Therapeutics	26	Surgery	104
Pharmacy	12	Obstetrics	104

Medical Jurisprudence	16	Operative Gynecology	26
Nervous Diseases	12	Eye and Ear	26
Principles of Medicine	26	Nose and Throat	26
Practice	78	Physical Diagnosis	26
Pathology	52	College/Hospital Clinics	312
Histological Lab	52	Total	898

FOURTH YEAR HOURS

Practice	78	Medical Jurisprudence	16
Pathology	52	Nervous Diseases	12
Surgery	104	College Clinics	260
Obstetrics	104	Eye and Ear	26
Operative Gynecology	26	Nose and Throat	26
Hospital Clinics	104	Total	808

The college's circular letter in 1904 estimated the cost of four years' reading, including annual sessions of twenty-seven weeks each, in four different college years. By purchasing a scholarship ticket for $250, a student could attend all four years, including any necessary repeats. In addition, the graduation fee was twenty-five dollars; book purchases averaged about twenty dollars; room and board, one hundred dollars; washing, eighteen dollars; hospital ticket, five dollars; and incidentals, fifteen dollars. The total cost of a full four years of medical education, according to the college, ranged from $722 to $1,074.[32]

The 1907–08 bulletin detailed the purchase of land at 630 West Sixth Street adjoining the sixty-bed Seton Hospital (formerly Presbyterian Hospital) belonging to the Sisters of Charity, on which the trustees of the college intended to erect a modern college building. Plans called for a five-story building with a bridge connecting to the hospital. Seton Hospital had twenty-four ward beds, thirty-six private rooms, two operating rooms, and a free dispensary open every day but Sunday from 8:00 to 10:30 in the morning. The hospital also cared for the "outdoor" medical cases as well as maternity cases in the home.[33]

When opened two years later, the new building contained a students' room, lavatory, and storeroom on the first floor; a large (125-seat) auditorium, offices, and library on the second floor; laboratories for physiology, histology, pathology, and bacteriology on the third floor; an anatomical and surgical amphitheater with seats for ninety students, a museum containing thirty-five complete skeletons for teaching, an operating amphitheater seating seventy, and a bridge connecting to Seton Hospital on the fourth floor; and a chemical laboratory and a dissecting room on the fifth floor. According to the college faculty, "it fully answers the demands modern medicine exacts from its devotees, being equipped most lavishly with everything necessary in the way of facilities to teach young people the latest and most advanced methods in the science and art of medicine."[34]

The institute's original library of several thousand volumes had been destroyed in the 1869 fire. Replacing this loss was slow. As late as 1909, the college reported a "working library" of only five hundred volumes, available to students two afternoons each week. Not until the construction of the new college adjoining Seton Hospital was space specifically devoted to library needs. By then, the library contained a thousand volumes with a reading room supplied with seventy-five eclectic, homeopathic, and regular journals. Students could use the reading room at stated periods during the term and a librarian was available twice a week. Students also had access to the public library and the medical library of the Cincinnati Hospital.[35] In addition, they could use the collection of eclecticana in the Lloyd Library, located in a newly constructed facility a few doors from the college. Its twenty thousand volumes, a herbarium that comprised thirty thousand species, and a large mycological collection of four thousand specimens represented a valuable research collection available to students and faculty.[36]

By 1911, the faculty had expanded the educational program to four years of graded course work, or 4,046 hours. This included 1,426 hours of didactic lectures, 1,390 hours of laboratory work, and 1,230 hours of clinics in Seton Hospital. The faculty graded students on daily recitations, written quizzes, and a final examination. Through all of this, the two key concepts for eclectic medicine were *specific medication* and *family practice*.[37] One hundred major and 250 minor operations were performed in the college operating amphitheater; five thousand dispensary patients were treated annually; and every student attended a minimum of six obstetric cases. In addition, each student administered at least one general anesthetic; attended lectures on clinical psychiatry at Longview Hospital; and took a course of instruction that included lectures, operations, bedside instruction, and autopsies at the Cincinnati General Hospital. Since college faculty was not represented on the staff of the Cincinnati Hospital, students worked under the supervision of a regular physician.[38]

Student Profile

Until the 1920s, student files at the college were sketchy, consisting of little more than an index card listing the student's name and home address, an Ohio certification number, the name of the school from which the student transferred, the years in attendance at EMC, and the student's graduation date. Seldom were there letters of correspondence or other materials.[39] The files after 1920 are more complete, including a new admission form that required the full name, address, class applied for, race, nationality, religion, date and place of birth, name and occupation of father or guardian, names of high schools and colleges attended (with dates), names of medical colleges to which applications for admission had been made and that were still pending, identification of any previous enrollment in any medical school, two character certificates, and a photograph. The form was consistent with most other schools.[40]

Students of native-born parents were typically sons of eclectic physicians, ministers, merchants, shop foremen, and insurance salesmen. Many had transferred from colleges and universities such as Indiana University, the University of Cincinnati, Xavier College, Bowling Green State College, Notre Dame, and Ohio State University where they had enrolled in a two-year premedical program.[41] In a few instances where brothers enrolled, they usually came from a medical family; and women students were almost always daughters of eclectic physicians. Sons and daughters of physicians tended to have greater academic difficulties, with a smaller than usual percentage graduating. It was not uncommon for a son to withdraw because of poor grades and a daughter to withdraw due to an illness such as neurasthenia.[42]

Parents desiring a son or daughter to enroll at EMC understood all too well the influence that alumni had on the admission decision. For example, a physician from Hackensack, New Jersey, wrote dean Byron Nellans regarding a student the college had declined to admit. "Please, do not misunderstand me, I do not want to send to *our college* inferior material or incompetents, but I am deeply concerned about the situation of the Eclectic Physicians in this State." Fearing the loss of representation on the State Board of Medical Examiners (mixed board) because of the declining numbers of graduates and also because of the inability of any of the existing eclectic schools to obtain class-A rankings from the American Medical Association's Council on Medical Education, he implored Nellans to take a risk with the young man. "May I add," he wrote, "this family is going to send him to study in Europe if we do not accept him; finance is not an obstacle; but I would like to hold him here and have him as one of our group, if you can take him in." He concluded by telling Nellans of the effort and personal sacrifices he had made to "keep alive" the Eclectic Medical Society of New Jersey. "I have no other reason otherwise, but the constant welfare and future of our Cause." Nellans accepted the student.[43]

DISCRIMINATION

Despite waves of immigrants that poured through New York harbor in the nineteenth century, most colleges and universities remained the private reserve of white, Anglo-Saxon, Protestant America. Liberal admission policies notwithstanding, these institutions served as the portal to the nation's managerial and professional positions. By the early twentieth century, however, academic administrators were voicing alarm at the changing ethnic and religious composition of their student body. For example, Jewish students who attended colleges and universities prior to the 1890s practiced Reform Judaism and came from families that had emigrated to the United States from Germany during the first half of the nineteenth century. By contrast, those who swelled the ranks of colleges in the early 1900s came principally from southern and eastern Europe and observed a more traditional orthodoxy. Poorer and culturally distinct from the German Jews, these new emigrants faced a more hostile environment than their predecessors.[44]

Nicholas Murray Butler, who succeeded Seth Low as president of Columbia University, discovered that the student mix had changed as the city's Jewish population took advantage of the secondary-school system and low college tuition. Recognizing that universities were "gatekeepers" to the professions and, wanting Columbia to become a premier national institution, Butler introduced a set of new admission policies intended to limit enrollment to "a fraction of those meeting the stated entrance requirements."[45] Unlike Harvard and other Ivy League schools whose admission policies were explicit in their restriction of Jews, Columbia chose a more circuitous ratiocination, but one that produced similar results. As part of its admissions materials, Columbia required information on the personal background of each applicant—place of birth and religious affiliation; father's name, place of birth, and occupation; mother's maiden name and place of birth; any name changes of family members; school activities, honors, prizes. This elaborate eight-page form, along with a required photograph, letters of recommendation (including one from a school principal), grades in course subjects, and personal interview, gave college admissions officers the information needed to restrict admittances to those with the most desirable characteristics.[46] In addition, Columbia screened applicants using a test to determine the "general mental ability" of the candidate. According to Dean Herbert E. Hawkes, "most Jews, especially those of the more objectionable type, have not had the home experiences which enable them to pass these tests as successfully as the average native American boy." Those judged least assimilated were denied admission.[47]

By 1921, the percentage of Jewish students at Columbia had declined from 40 to 22 percent. Butler's decision to make Columbia more selective fit a much larger pattern of actions taken by other elite Eastern schools in the 1920s. This phenomenon, as explained by Thomas Bender in his New York Intellect (1987), was "Protestant at its core [and] was at once forward-looking in its commitment to professional standards and reactionary in its fears of immigration as subversive of the values of Anglo-American civilization."[48]

Similar attitudes affected professional schools. The concerns regarding the high number of Jewish applicants to medical schools, for example, tended to focus on the fear of the profession becoming more of a money-making business, a difference of ethical viewpoints, a resentment against the admission of immigrant children, and the need for schools to represent a more balanced population. "Since training cost much more than tuition fees," wrote Marcia Graham Synnott in The Half-Opened Door (1979), "every Jewish applicant admitted to medical school was seen as another expensively subsidized competitor of the native-born American. And every Jewish doctor allegedly took a position away from a native American doctor."[49]

In 1918, Columbia Medical School became the first professional school to adopt a selective admissions policy. Prior to 1918, Jewish students comprised about half of each entering class. By 1924, the percentage had declined to between 18 and 20 percent and would continue to decline to 12 percent by the Second World War.[50] In Long Island Hospital Medical College, Jewish students comprised 80 percent of the 1926 entering class and only 45 percent of the 1928 class. At New York Homeopathic Medical College, the ratio was 69 percent Jews in the 1929–30 entering class but only 34 percent in 1934.

Clearly, discrimination existed, but pressures from the Association of American Medical Colleges and the Council on Medical Education also affected medical school admission policies. While the statistics indicate a significant decrease in the number of Jews admitted to medical schools, the total number of medical students also declined during this period as part of the overall reduction in the number of medical schools and the increase in admission standards. The declining number of medical schools and reduced numbers of medical students caused many school administrators to seek better balances between the sons and daughters of older Americans and the children of new immigrants.

The Jewish community in nineteenth-century Cincinnati had been central European in descent and modest in size compared to communities on the East Coast. Characterized by strong social interaction with the Christian majority, the city's Jews practiced their religion freely, played a prominent role in the economic and professional life of the community, and were immensely loyal to the city. Cincinnati was the oldest Jewish community west of the Alleghenies. Between 1816, when the first known Jewish settler arrived in the city of about six thousand inhabitants, and 1836, the year marking the opening of the first synagogue on Sixth Street and Broadway, the Jewish population began to coalesce out of the waves of new immigrants from Great Britain and Germany. By 1850, the community boasted the first Jewish hospital in America and by 1854 its first newspaper; and by the end of the Civil War, Cincinnati was home to several synagogues, including a Moorish-style building on Plum Street, opposite the city's leading Catholic and Unitarian churches. Although the acknowledged home of Reform Judaism, Cincinnati in the post–Civil War era would witness immigration from Russia, Poland, and Romania and, with it, the beginnings of a distinctive new orthodoxy that would reshape the community's character.[51]

Many immigrant families, frustrated in attempts to enroll their sons in the more restrictive East Coast medical schools, chose instead to enroll them in unapproved medical schools, "taking a chance on [their] becoming licensed to practice."[52] For young men of Jewish heritage, the eclectic college in Cincinnati became a safe haven during the 1920s and 1930s. The majority of them, sons of immigrants living in New York and New Jersey, were outstanding students, hard workers, and anxious that the AMA's classification of the college not stand in the way of their professional opportunities. The parents of these students were themselves immigrants from Italy, Austria-Hungary, Germany, Russia, and Lithuania. Fathers typically included clothiers, furriers, fruit produce dealers, grocers, merchants, contractors, dress manufacturers, tailors, dye workers, manufacturers of soft drinks or cosmetics, and realtors. Of the students, a good number had transferred from Long Island University, New York University, and the University of Alabama, all of which offered a two-year program in premedical education.[53]

LICENSURE AND STUDENT TRANSFERS

Throughout the eighteenth and early nineteenth centuries, doctors who served apprenticeships were able to declare themselves physicians by virtue of their membership in local medical societies. Later, diplomas from almost any type of medical school, regardless of standing or particular philosophy, fulfilled the legal requirements for entrance into the profession. State legislation designed to raise standards through the passage of stringent licensing examinations developed slowly and against the judgment of a nation whose elected representatives showed contempt for the presumed elitist implications of such regulations. Nevertheless, increasingly enlightened efforts among reformers brought nineteen state medical boards into existence by 1878 and twenty-six by 1891.

Between 1833 and 1868, Ohio chose not to regulate medical practice. After 1868, the state required doctors to present a diploma from a medical school or a certificate from a county medical society to practice. This law remained in force until 1880 when it was revised to require that the diploma be issued after attendance at two full sessions of at least twelve weeks' duration. Five years later, in an effort to tighten the law, the legislature stipulated that the diploma be from a "reputable" medical school. Sadly, actual practice veered far short of legislative intent. In 1890, a survey undertaken by the Illinois State

Board of Health revealed that the Ohio law had not been enforced. Not until 1896 did the Ohio legislature follow the lead of thirty-one other states in establishing a state board of medical registration and examination. Even so, the law recognized either a diploma from a medical school or proof of ten years of continuous practice for a license to be issued. Not until 1900 did the law require candidates to pass an examination in all branches of medicine.

Abraham Flexner viewed state boards as instruments of medical reconstruction in the United States. By enforcing preliminary educational requirements, establishing minimal standards for medical school facilities, and examining graduates for licensure, they became the single most important quality-control point in the medical education system. The license of the state was, under ideal conditions, "a guarantee of knowledge, education, and skill." For boards to do their duty, they needed to be properly constituted and equipped with legal powers to enforce their decision making. To the extent that they were unwilling or legally unable to overturn decisions and actions of medical schools, they served only to exacerbate a low-grade product. Flexner concluded that "far-reaching legislative changes" were essential if state boards were to play the part assigned to them. Short of that, medicine would remain in hands soiled by ignorance, incompetence, and commercialism.[54]

Nationally, medical licensure in 1923 was in the control of forty-nine separate jurisdictions, each legally independent of all others and acting under forty-nine different acts that provided for fifty-seven separate licensing boards. Thirty-eight states authorized a composite board, which meant that each of the principal schools of medicine (regular, homeopathic, eclectic, physio-medical) had representation. In five states, a single board consisting only of regulars controlled medical licensure; in the remaining six states the practice laws provided for separate boards for each of the principal schools. In seven states having composite boards, representation was extended to osteopaths and special provision was made for examining so-called drugless practitioners.[55] Forty-five states required some level of premedical education for licensure; thirty-three gave their boards power to refuse recognition to low-grade medical colleges; and four made no provision in their practice acts for applicants even to be graduates of a medical college.[56]

Reciprocity was a complex set of interlocking relationships—some collegial, many conflicting, others unduly complicated. Notwithstanding these differences, reciprocity implied the exchange of the courtesies of licensure from one state to another. A physician from Indiana seeking a license to practice in Ohio had to meet the same qualifications expected of a physician in Ohio at the date of the Indianan's original registration. Reciprocity consisted of two classes: Condition Number One endorsed the license of another state issued on the basis of a state board examination; Condition Number Two endorsed a license issued by another state on diploma registration. This latter condition usually applied to physicians who had graduated prior to 1900. While some states issued Condition Number One licenses only, others issued both, and some issued none at all.[57]

Loosely administered, reciprocity provided an open door through which unqualified candidates obtained registration in other states. Some boards wisely reserved the right to reject candidates who did not possess satisfactory credentials and others simply required applicants to have engaged in practice for at least one year in the state where the original license was granted before considering reciprocity. In 1912, the Ohio medical colleges having the highest failures before other state boards were Cleveland-Pulte Medical College (homeopathic) with 23 percent and EMC with 25 percent.[58]

Since a large number of EMC's graduates were from New York and returned there to practice, the licensing regulations determined by the regents of the University of New York remained a baseline for the college's admission and graduation requirements. In 1914, a school could be registered with the regents if it was legally incorporated and owned apparatus and equipment worth at least fifty thousand dollars. The regents also expected each school to require of its candidates that they be at least twenty-one years of age, of good moral character, and have studied medicine for not less than four school years of seven months each. Equally important, every medical school had to require that its matriculants show evidence of a general preliminary education equivalent to at least four years of high school and eight years of elementary preparation; no allowance was given to any period of study taken in a nonaccredited medical school. Unlike other state boards, the New York regents refused to give advanced standing to the graduates of liberal arts colleges, dentistry, veterinary, pharmacy, or other professional and technical schools.[59]

In 1914, the regents gave class-A status to sixty-four fully registered medical schools, among them the Eclectic Medical College of Cincinnati. The regents also accredited twenty-six schools for three years only, thirteen for two years, and four for one year. This explains the not-uncommon transfer of students to EMC from schools that had been accredited with one, two, or only three years of professional work.[60] These included the University of Alabama School of Medicine in Tuscaloosa; Dartmouth Medical School in Hanover, New Hampshire; University of North Carolina School of Medicine in Chapel Hill; Wake Forest College School of Medicine, North Carolina; University of North Dakota School of Medicine, Grand Forks; University of South Dakota School of Medicine, Vermilion; University of Utah School of Medicine, Salt Lake City; and West Virginia University School of Medicine, Morgantown. A large number of EMC's transfer students came from two schools: University of Alabama School of Medicine and West Virginia University School of Medicine.[61]

Unlike the better allopathic schools, which took seriously the higher admission standards demanded by the Association of American Medical Colleges and the AMA's Council on Medical Education, EMC seemed content to serve as a second or third option for students with "honorable dismissals" (dismissal for academic reasons rather than behavioral problems, cheating, etc.).[62] It was not unusual for students to transfer into EMC with grades of E, or the equivalent "conditioned" (50–59 percent grade point average), or with F, meaning failure (0–49 percent grade point average). Dean W. J. Means of the Ohio State University College of Medicine wrote John K. Scudder in 1915 of a student who had attended the 1913–14 session but whose grades were too low to allow him to repeat his freshman year. He advised Scudder that, should EMC matriculate him, it should be as a beginning freshman. "He is not a bad sort of a fellow but it is the consensus of opinion among our teachers that he is not capable of mastering the fundamental sciences of a medical course." Scudder accepted the student, who graduated in the class of 1919.[63]

One student transferred from the University of Cincinnati Medical College in 1918 with three Cs, three Ds, and two Fs. Another transferred into the sophomore year from Loyola University School of Medicine, Chicago, in 1919 with six Ds, one F, and one C in his freshman year and six Fs in his sophomore year. Other students transferred in their junior and even senior years with low or failing grades.[64] A student refused advancement to the junior class of New York Homeopathic Medical College and prohibited from repeating his sophomore year (since he already had repeated his freshman year) was accepted into EMC and graduated in 1922. Another transferred from the same homeopathic college having failed his fourth year and his re-examination. Yet another student completed his freshman year with a combination of Fs and Cs and his sophomore year with a total of nine Fs before transferring to EMC and graduating in the class of 1922.[65] Similar records exist for student transfers from New York University and Bellevue Hospital Medical College, George Washington University Medical School, and the University of Cincinnati. One transfer from the University of Cincinnati carried five Ds, four Fs, and two Es.[66]

While family physicians and ministers typically provided uncritical letters of support, tough and starkly honest evaluations came from science faculty in the students' premedical curriculum. Chairman and zoologist Raymond C. Osburn of Ohio State University remarked about one former student: "He seemed to me not at all brilliant, but rather gifted with persistence, determination and the ability to work steadily. . . . If you are after brilliant young men of the research type, I cannot recommend him, but if you prefer the honest, dependable, conscientious type who will do his whole duty without making any 'splurge' in the medical profession I can recommend him to you on this basis."[67] When Dean John N. Simpson of the West Virginia University Medical School commented on a student seeking to transfer to EMC after having failed half of his work, the dean reported that the young man had "nothing against him other than poor scholarship." Undeterred by the letter, EMC accepted the student who repeated his freshman year and graduated in 1928.[68]

One particular transfer case in 1919 is worth noting. John K. Scudder received a letter from a department chair at the Detroit College of Medicine and Surgery, an alumnus of EMC. The letter referenced a student dismissed for scholastic reasons and who was attempting to transfer to EMC. According to the department chair, the student "has quite a bad record here scholastically and also by reputation. By some of the men under whom he worked he is considered mentally and morally below par." He further stated that the faculty who had taught him were "unanimous in refusing to further consider his case [because of] poor scholarship and his persistence in making false representations." Despite this negative information, Scudder admitted the student to EMC and he, too, graduated in 1922.[69]

Transfer students did better in their studies at EMC. No doubt for many parents, the college represented the medical school of last chance for sons and daughters who had done poorly at other schools. EMC students on average obtained a 10 to 15 percentage point break in their grades. In most instances, this level of grade inflation sufficed to ensure graduation.

In the fourteen years between 1925 and 1939, the college matriculated a total of 414 students. During those years, the six states that contributed the largest number of students to the college were Ohio, 136; New York, 101; New Jersey, 54; Kentucky, 29; Pennsylvania, 21; and Illinois, 11. Students from New York and New Jersey averaged 44.2 percent in each of the graduating classes.[70]

Of the 414 matriculants in this fourteen-year period, 349 started as freshmen, 34 transferred in as sophomores, 19 came as juniors, and 12 as seniors. The largest number of freshmen came from the University of Cincinnati (43), Ohio State University (26), New York University (26), Xavier College in Cincinnati (22), Long Island University (14), Columbia University (13), the University of Alabama (13), and the College of the City of New York (10). Sophomores came principally from New York Homeopathic Medical School (8) and George Washington University (5). The largest number of juniors transferred in from the Long Island College Hospital (9), while seniors came from the Hahnemann Medical College of Chicago (8). The remaining students came in smaller numbers from an assortment of other schools.

Of the 414 matriculants, sixty-three failed to graduate; nineteen withdrew without giving a reason, eleven because of poor grades; eleven transferred to other colleges (the largest number in 1936–37 following the board's decision to close the college); and ten withdrew because of illness and nine for financial reasons.

DISCIPLINARY ISSUES

Not surprisingly, some of the more difficult disciplinary problems concerned the sons and daughters of alumni. Perhaps these students expected preferential treatment from the college because of their parents, or perhaps they enrolled because of parental pressure and not from personal choice. In any case, an inordinate number were dismissed because of poor scholarship or, worse, because of cheating. One pair of brothers who enrolled in the class of 1931–32 lasted only a year. While the record is not clear, it appears that the reason for their dismissal was a combination of cheating and poor grades. Rather than accept responsibility for their actions, they accused Dean Nellans of dismissing them because of feelings the dean allegedly harbored against their father when he was in school in 1922.[71] One of the brothers wrote T. D. Adlerman, M.D., of Brooklyn, New York, who was secretary of the National Eclectic Medical Association. Using as an excuse a letter from Alderman to the boy's father asking him to rejoin the association, the son proceeded to lay out his case to the secretary and threatened to cause trouble for the association and the college if the matter was not brought to a favorable conclusion.[72]

Another parent and physician wrote college treasurer C.W. Beaman complaining that his son had been disenrolled because of "a misdemeanor [presumably cheating] that involved more than half the class." Convinced that both Beaman and Nellans were "prejudiced against the boy," he determined not to appeal the ruling even though it resulted "in an irreparable wrong" to himself and his son. Instead, the father prepared a set of questions challenging the integrity of the faculty, their pedagogy and grading practices, and the relevance of the curriculum.[73] Beaman wrote back with an itemized response to the father's questions. His answers give insight into the faculty's teaching practices.[74]

> 1. Every teacher in the employment of the College with the exception of one, has years of teaching experience. They are employed to give an adequate and up-to-date course of study, and to grade without fear or favor. The Executive Committee of the Board of Trustees, has confidence in the ability and honesty of these teachers. From the many Faculty conferences, I am confident that no split hair decisions are made relative to the grades of any students.

> 2. Grades are based on the totality of a student's work, and his general attitude toward a given subject. The Administrative department has no reason to doubt the sincerity of a teacher in arriving at his conclusions. Opportunity is given to every student to appeal his case, but the executive department does not overrule a faculty member on the question of scholarship.

3. Any student cheating in his relation to the College, injures himself, more than he does the institution. That all cases of copying and cheating are not found out, is only too true, but if it were known, a severe penalty would be the result.

4. Every grade is on file, and no grade has been changed in the office, having been received over the signature of the instructor. We should like to have proof that such an incident occurred.

5. There are recognized rules which govern College instruction, both academic and professional, which permit the student to make up work, where failure and conditions are within certain limits. When the student's record of failures and conditions exceeds this limit, he loses this right. The student knows this, when he enters the College, and if properly prepared, he should make the grades required.

6. Time alone can answer this question, as to how much the truths taught today, will be acceptable twenty-five years hence. However, grades are based on current medical knowledge.

7. Independence of thought should always be encouraged, but there is a limit to this. The student is required to follow a given text, and to be familiar with the truth as set forth. The independence of his thoughts must not interfere with his ability to answer according to his instruction. . . . Some students, unfortunately, glory in the fact that they differ from the standard course of instruction, but no teacher can evaluate their opinions. This should be left until after they have gotten out of school, and have developed the truth of their ideas.

8. Every thinking man should encourage flexibility of thought. Outside of mathematics, there are few things in a curriculum that are inflexible. However, it is the instructor who must determine the degree of flexibility, and not the student.

9. A teacher is selected because of his known reputation for knowledge in his given department. If he proves incompetent, it will not be long before he will be out of a job, and a better man employed.

10. Qualified teachers educated in an Eclectic College will always have precedence over those, from any other source. We are doing all in our power to either acquire or train such men for positions in the college.

Then there were cases that simply defied resolution. In January 1934, Dean Nellans informed a graduate of the class of 1910 that his son could not return for the sophomore year because of poor grades in four major subjects. The son had already spent one year at Miami University and two years at Ohio State University before transferring as a freshman to EMC. The decision of the promotions committee, wrote Nellans, had been based "entirely upon scholarship." The dean went on to comment that the fact that the young man "was caught with a 'pony' in the final examination in anatomy had little if any bearing upon the action." Nellans urged the father to enroll the son in a college of liberal arts to obtain a baccalaureate degree and then, perhaps, to begin again with his medical studies.[75]

In responding to the dean's letter, the father first accused Nellans of deliberately delaying the refund of his son's tuition and lab breakage fees.[76] He then wrote Frank J. Andress, M.D., his son's chemistry professor, complaining that the "conditioned" grade given his son had been made on the basis of improper calculations of the test scores.[77] Andress responded with a full explanation of how the grade had been derived.[78] The parent then accused Nellans of alleging things about his son that were "without truth or foundation." In particular, he accused Nellans and the faculty of having stigmatized his son with dishonesty because a pony was in his possession at the time of the examination. Such a claim, the doctor wrote Nellans, "is not only a discredit to you but . . . to the Institution of which you are the Secretary."[79]

Taking matters into his own hands, the parent questioned the son's comrades, who gave assurances that the son had not used the pony during the examination. Convinced that his son's reputation had been maligned, the father demanded that the college provide affidavits establishing the fact that his son had been caught using a pony during the examination. "We do not send our young sons and daughters to college," he wrote Nellans, "to have their ambitions crucified upon the altars of those Professors who place more stress upon having them assuming an 'attitude' of worship at their feet than they do of learning the subject matter at hand. We send our sons and daughters to college to fit them to proficiently occupy some useful place in society and not to have their pride insulted by gross accusations of dishonesty in the class room which are false and unwarranted."[80]

Nellans tried unsuccessfully to assure the father that the faculty had the highest regard for his son and that the college's decision to dismiss him was based entirely on his poor scholarship rather than on any accusation of cheating or dishonesty. While he had been caught with a pony in the examination room, at no time had the faculty accused him of actually using it. Nellans concluded by saying that he held no personal animosity against the young man and was confident he would make a success in life. "I frankly pledge you my earnest desire to be of service in planning your son's future."[81]

None of Nellan's explanations were accepted by the parent, who accused the faculty of duplicity and returned his son's certificate of dismissal as something "unwarranted, unjust and vicious." The college files do not contain information on the final resolution of the case except a note scribbled at the bottom of the father's last letter to Nellans indicating that the "certificate of dismissal was not endorsed."[82]

Another parent, himself an eclectic graduate practicing in Wapakoneta, Ohio, wrote Nellans on behalf of his son who had been dismissed for poor scholarship.

> From what I see of other graduates both from our school and competitive schools and having had [my son] with me in Hospitals and helping even in Obstetrics and minor operations I know that the boy would be a credit to our school, and feeling as I do could there be some way of allowing him to continue as a sophomore next year and then if he cant carry the work fire him. Owing to our having very intimate friends in St. Louis and all of us having graduated from the Eclectic we have considered these schools for him above all others, and now to lose out in our own school it would be rather tough, as stated in our conversation on phone. . . . So won't you please see some of these prof. in person and intercede to allow him to complete this years course, even if conditioned and make him take the exams, in the fall. I feel that he will be successful if graduated [sic].[83]

Ever polite, Nellans advised the unhappy parent that sickness and unexcused absences from class had dampened his son's prospects for success at the college. "Your son is more than mentally capable of passing the courses," Nellans wrote, but "the big thing is his attendance, and the apparent lack of application." The student returned and repeated his freshman year but later transferred to Ohio State University Medical School.[84]

One particularly disgruntled parent, an eclectic physician from Troy, Ohio, whose son had lasted only one session in 1932–33, complained that Nellans had "thwarted [his] son's future prospects; and wish you to bear in mind that you surely will 'Reap what you have sown.' Could give you more in detail, but in time you will gain that knowledge." In closing, he noted the school's lack of recognition by the Association of American Medical Colleges and the Council on Medical Education and indicated that his own retribution would be correspondingly harsh.[85]

CHAPTER FOUR

Student Life

THE CIVIL WAR left Cincinnati outdistanced by St. Louis and Chicago, but it remained a dynamic confluence of railroads, river barges, and entrepreneurs united by money, trade, and politics. With its markets diminished by the aggressive power of the Louisville and Nashville Railroad to the east, the city responded in the 1870s and 1880s with festive industrial expositions intended to bring new life to its commerce and industry. This, combined with the Cincinnati Southern Railway's new markets in the South, resulted in a renewed era of industrial vigor. By 1890, output of industrial products from the Queen City had risen to $110 million, requiring a workforce of more than 8,400. Although Cincinnati reluctantly turned over its title as "pork packer of the West" to Chicago, it continued to produce more than half of the country's carriages and wagons. Similarly, the soap-making and brewing industries stepped up production, the latter producing more than a million and a half barrels annually. Boots and shoes, men's clothing, malt liquors, and machine-shop products were all manufactured in Cincinnati.[1]

At the turn of the century, Cincinnatians proudly claimed that Vine Street rivaled Broadway in New York City and Market Street in San Francisco. There one could find concert halls, shooting galleries, bowling alleys, burlesque, and saloons selling twenty-one glasses of beer for a dollar. Along Vine Street were no less than 113 saloons, including Atlantic Garden, Pacific Gardens, Kisel's Concert Hall, Schuman's, and Weber's. Some twenty-five pictures hung on the walls of the Stagg saloon, but the painting most prized by patrons was *The Sirens*, depicting three nymphs lolling by the sea. Vine Street was known for its pilsners, bourbons, and German food that was both inexpensive and plentiful—from steamed dumplings and sausages to potato pancakes, kidney soup, hamhocks, and sauerbraten. Of course, the street also sported beggars, trollops, con men, and drummers.[2]

By the turn of the century, Cincinnati, with a population of 325,000, was home to four of the ten medical schools in Ohio—the Medical College of Ohio, the Eclectic Medical Institute, Miami Medical College, and Pulte Medical College. Board for medical students averaged three to five dollars per week, with tuition at the two regular schools set at $125 and $130 respectively, while EMI and Pulte charged seventy-five dollars. The session for the Medical College of Ohio ran from September 8 through June 1; that of Miami Medical College from October 1 through June 1; EMI from September 19 through April 21; and Pulte Medical College from September 27 through May 2.[3]

EARLY MATRICULANTS

In his essay on the making of an eclectic, Ronald L. Numbers recounted the life of Joseph M. McElhinney, who arrived in Cincinnati in October 1854 "carrying his trunk, carpet sack, pistol, and books." After finding a place to board for $2.25 a week, he and 279 other students (including sixteen women) attended lectures at EMI, where dean Joseph Rodes Buchanan and a faculty of seven professors held forth on reform practice. Six days a week, he walked to the four-story institute where he listened to special instruction on phrenology and mesmerism, observed surgical operations in the school's amphitheater, labored in the dissection room, and attended Newton's Clinical Institute. Since McElhinney had not served an apprenticeship prior to attending EMI, he listed the school as his preceptor—a not uncommon practice in the day. He attended only one sixteen-week session instead of the preferred two and returned to Newport, in southeastern Ohio, where he set up practice without having received a degree.[4] As William Norwood observed in his *Medical Education in the United States Before the Civil War* (1944), only about one-third of the matriculants in this period ever graduated.[5] This explains why it is more important in the nineteenth century to know the total number of matriculants in a medical school than count the number of graduates, since most were likely to enter practice. By 1886, EMI had 8,888 matriculants, 2,802 of whom graduated.[6]

Like students today, after the last class on Friday, thoughts turned to relaxation, even though classes continued on Saturday. Among the pleasures of Cincinnati were "stag" banquets attended by both students and faculty. At the Hotel Metropole and similar establishments, students gathered for impromptu toasts, friendly advice from their professors, impersonations, songs, and poetry.[7] At one soirée, eighty students, faculty, and guests met for vocal and instrumental music, followed by humor aimed at regulars, homeopaths, and toasts by Thomas Vaughan Morrow (known by students and colleagues as the "Steam Engine" of EMI), James H. Oliver (the "Galvanic Battery" of reform), Benjamin L. Hill (the "Bone and Muscle" of the faculty), Ichabod Gibson Jones (the "Flower of the Flock"), and Joseph R. Buchanan (the "Head-piece" of the faculty). Along with farcical songs that included mock fights with old-school doctors and their prescriptions of calomel, Buchanan led the gathering in singing the "Song of the Reformers," which he had written for the occasion and sang to the tune of the "Star-Spangled Banner."

Song of the Reformers

Come rouse up, Reformers! the night has gone by!
    Through the blue vault of Heaven the sunlight is beaming,
The Clouds have departed, and beneath a clear sky,
    Our Flag far and wide is now gallantly streaming.
No longer the lonely and buffeted few—
    We march as an army—united and true.
Then rouse up, Reformers! the night has gone by—
    And our flag, far and wide, is now floating on high.

We battle against the dread armies of Death!
    And to God alone look for the biddings of duty;
Our oracles are not a frail mortal's breath—
    We kneel before Nature and worship her beauty.
And we march to a victory, bloodless and blessed!
'Tis to conquer Disease and relieve the distressed.
    Then rouse up, Reformers! the night has gone by,
And our flag, far and wide, is now floating on high.

We've broken our fetters—they are trampled in dust,
    We've crushed every barrier in our career;

And conquer we will—and conquer we must!
    For the might of Jehovah shall go with us here.
Then on! like the Templar Knights, valiant of old,
    Yet gentle and graceful, and winning as bold.
Cry onward! Reformers! the night has gone by,
    And our flag, far and wide, is now floating on high.

Away with your systems of falsehood and wrong,
    That only were made for the dullard and craven;
When we battle for truth we are mighty and strong,
    And we dare to be free as the wild winds of Heaven!
Our watchword's Progression! our day is before us;
    And the Sun of Reform has but dawned on its glories!
Cry onward, Reformers! the night has gone by,
    And our flag, far and wide, is now floating on high![8]

Buchanan, as facile with the pen as he was with his tongue, also contributed a poem on "The Good Time Coming," sung by a Dr. Sells at another college banquet in 1850. One particular stanza referred to

Senseless rivalries of schools,
Shall not make their followers fools,
    In the good time coming.
Lancets shall be lost in rust,
And calomel be worthless dust,
    In the good time coming.[9]

Between Joseph McElhinney's time and the late nineteenth century, the experiences of students at EMI did not dramatically change. Classes were still held six days of the week and continued to be principally didactic. The curriculum, while less idiosyncratic, remained fixated on eclecticism's decidedly protestant view of itself. By 1870, Scudder's system of specific medication had entered the curriculum and reform practice became less a matter of substituting vegetable for mineral medicines and more a matter of small amounts of specific medication.

WOMEN AND MINORITIES

The eclectics were among the earliest to accept women into their medical colleges at Worcester, Syracuse, Rochester, and Cincinnati, and, like homeopaths, they took pride in proclaiming that women enjoyed the same advantages as male students. The National Eclectic Medical Association endorsed coeducation in 1852 and by the time of the Civil War, nearly three hundred women had graduated from its various schools. The eclectics, according to Alexander Wilder, had admitted women not just to their schools but to equal favor in their medical societies. However laudable the intent, Wilder's observation missed the mark by a considerable degree.[10]

As for the regulars, after Geneva Medical College in New York tested the troubled waters of women's medical education in 1847 by admitting Elizabeth Blackwell, they concluded that women were out of their proper sphere and, with minor exceptions, closed their ranks to women physicians for another thirty years. Not surprisingly, EMI found it easier to avoid the stigma of feminism and unorthodox practice by acknowledging women's "natural" limitations and urging them to seek more satisfying work in nursing and midwifery. The realm of medicine, remarked eclectic George W. L. Bickley, M.D., "with its stark immediacy to death, disease, and social impurities," tended to "unsex the woman physician in a perverse and dehumanizing way."[11] Bickley's comment was soon followed by an announcement in August 1857 that EMI would no longer admit female students. "While we do not oppose the medical education of ladies," remarked the editor of the *Eclectic Medical Journal*, the school's official organ, "we would advise all such students to avail themselves of the ample opportunities now afforded them at medical schools established for their exclusive benefit."[12] From 1853 until the teach-out of matriculants in 1859, the institute graduated twenty-six female physicians (see appendix).

Although EMI closed its doors to women, other eclectic schools remained open, a situation that, as Regina Morantz-Sanchez observed, only exacerbated the bitter feelings between medical orthodoxy and sectarian medicine.[13] Equally important, five regular schools for women were founded between 1850 and 1882, which relieved regular colleges, their faculty, and trustees from the embarrassment of having to refuse women applicants. Arguing that women deserved to have their own colleges to protect their natural modesty and offer subjects more at-tuned to their sex, the newly founded American Medical Association was able to sidestep public criticism of these fledgling schools. Never-theless, public and professional ostracism tracked both the graduates of these second-class schools and their teaching faculty. Lacking re-spected teachers and faced with haphazard equipment and clinical experience, many women chose foreign study in Zurich and Paris to acquire the education and clinical opportunities denied them at home. Notwithstanding their efforts, on returning to the United States, few found lucrative practices.[14]

Beginning in the 1870s, along with Boston University Homeo-pathic College, the Cleveland Homeopathic Hospital College, the University of Michigan Homeopathic Medical College, Hahnemann Medical College in Chicago, the Homeopathic Medical Department of the State University of Iowa, and a small number of regular schools, EMI reversed itself and admitted women. From 1874 until its final closing, EMI graduated a total of ninety-nine women physicians.[15]

One of EMI's more outstanding women alumni was Louise East-man, who graduated from EMI in 1898. She practiced for thirty-five years, maintaining offices at her residence at 4329 Beach Hill Ave-nue, Northside, and in downtown Cincinnati. A lifelong Republican, she advocated women's suffrage and the corset, was president of the Cincinnati Eclectic Maternity Society, and was a frequent speaker at the annual conventions of the National Eclectic Medical Asso-ciation.[16]

EMI declared itself open from the 1870s on to men and women who had reached the age of seventeen, but it chose not to solicit the matriculation of African American students, believing that "they can be better educated in institutions devoted exclusively to their race."[17] Notwithstanding this statement, EMI may well have graduated the first black physician in the United States. At least that is what John Uri Lloyd claimed. Although not clearly identifiable through alumni records, the individual may have been William R. Reynolds of Illinois, who graduated in the class of 1868. In a letter from Booker T. Washington to John Uri Lloyd, dated May 2, 1900, Washington thanked Lloyd for sharing the information.[18] Similarly, there is the possibility of other black students in class pictures in the 1890s. At least two class photographs exist in the archives of the Lloyd Library and Museum in Cincinnati that suggest this.

LATER MATRICULANTS

Students entering EMI in the 1890s might have felt a change in curricular expectations, but their lives continued much as before. A student's first impression of Cincinnati after arriving by rail in the autumn of 1895 was its smoky, sooty, and noisy appearance. Relieved of his baggage by a small delegation of upperclassmen, the freshman was introduced to a peculiar etiquette he would follow through his first year at EMI. Comments such as "Isn't he cute?" and "I wonder what drug firm he travels for?" and "Who left the gate open?" prepared the young medical student for the hazing that was about to commence.

After arriving at the college, he registered and received a list of possible rooms for lease on a weekly or monthly basis.[19] In the early days of the college, the faculty took special care to select suitable boarding for students in private houses to ensure a quiet environment for study, one reminiscent of home. For those of more limited means, the school treasurer procured rooms where students could board themselves, bringing their expenses below three dollars per week. By the 1890s, the student's typical habitat was a rooming house within blocks of the school where he rented a single room or shared one with one or more students. One of the choice places was the YMCA, a block from the school, where, for a small weekly fee, students obtained comfortable—albeit austere—furnishings for their school sessions. Into these sparse quarters, they brought clothes, books, sports gear, cigars and cigarettes, anatomical charts, and the occasional skull that served as an ashtray.

A new student's first full day at the college found him the center of attention, surrounded by sophomores ordering him to sing, prepare orations, or simply answer impertinent questions. Upperclassmen found sport introducing freshmen to the dissecting room, where they forced the newcomers to greet each cadaver and shake its hand.[20]

The only courtesy given the new student was by janitor "Uncle Ben" Hickman, who treated everyone as if he or she had been a lifetime resident of the city.[21] So pleased were students with the school's janitors that they were always remembered in later years. Uncle Ben worked for the school for twenty-nine years, and when he died on March 7, 1900, students and faculty attended his funeral and published resolutions of appreciation in the *Eclectic Medical Journal* and the *Medical Gleaner*.[22] In the class yearbook for 1911, the senior class gave a full-page portrait of the school's new genial janitor, George A. Baker, a Virginian known for his kindly disposition except when some "expectorator" marked his newly cleaned floors. Of course, the title of janitor was somewhat a misnomer, since Hickman, Baker, and their predecessors proved indispensable not only in maintaining the college premises but in "finding" suitable cadavers, storing them in brine vats in the basement, and eventually hauling them to the dissection rooms on the top floor. Janitors also supplemented their salary by connecting students with local vendors to supply food, laundry, mending, and an assortment of other amenities.[23]

Students fondly remembered their first day of classes when professor William E. Bloyer, dressed in a Prince Albert suit of black, mounted the lecture platform, bowed to the newly arrived students, and heartily welcomed them on behalf of the faculty. Armed with crayons, chalk, and an eraser, he proceeded to outline the scheme of instruction, "assuring all present that the information imparted would be sensible, practical and as accurate as possible; that, while it would be thorough and up-to-date, it was not intended to fritter away the valuable time of the student in seriously contemplating fads and fancies." In short, he told the class, "we propose to teach you medicine pure and simple, and that without any flummery, frills, flounces, or furbellows."[24]

John Uri Lloyd, the school's principal benefactor, was not without good counsel and fatherly advice. He drew attention to the dangers of the city and to its "gilded marble palaces of vice." Those who thought themselves free from the observation of friends and acquaintances and chose to indulge "in questionable practices, particularly in immoral conduct," would find that "the very walls will speak!"[25] Freshmen also received warm words of advice from Dean Frederick J. Locke, who, amid the din of street noise, attempted to ease the fears and uncertainties that consumed their thoughts on that first day.

Classes

Lectures began promptly at 7:30 each morning and students were required to be in their assigned seats and ready for class, including the much-hated daily quizzes.[26] Other than Thanksgiving and Christmas vacations, the calendar was punctuated by three special courses of lectures that lasted three weeks each in November, December, and January and five special lectures in January, February, March, and April. In

April, students took their examinations, followed by "Clinic Week," consisting of lectures and demonstrations in the specialties, internal medicine, and surgery and intended for the benefit of alumni who gathered annually to celebrate the graduation of a new class.[27]

Dissecting cadavers was grimly attended by each member of the class. It was the one occasion when smoking was not prohibited and where cheap imported cigars were considered perfume compared to the putrid smell of decaying bodies. Most students took to the work with considerable hesitation and the occasional female student had to be excused after crying and trembling from the experience. A neighbor once complained to police that students had "captured" a corpse and taken the body for dissection. When police entered the fourth-floor anatomy room, they found—through smoke, smarting eyes, and unhealthy fumes of formaldehyde—that the claim had been false and withdrew in haste from the students' "sanctum sanctorum."[28]

Beginning in the 1890s, the faculty began posting rules of conduct in the college's annual announcements. Students were expected to show proper decorum, including orderly conduct in the lecture rooms, laboratories, and halls; make no interruption in the classroom after the professor or lecturer entered; be in regular attendance in their assigned seats; and refrain from smoking (except in the dissection rooms) and defacing walls or furniture. Infringement of the rules subjected the student to a private or public reprimand, temporary suspension by the dean, or expulsion by the trustees.[29]

Tragedies inevitably struck one or two students each year, including nervous breakdown, tuberculosis, bankruptcy, family crisis, and even death. One student on the first day of classes learned by telegraph of his father's passing. His classmates saw him to the railway station as, despondent, he left to take over the family business. "We watched him go with deep sympathy in our hearts," wrote the class historian, "knowing that his dream of becoming a doctor had just been dashed.[30]

CLASS ANTICS

The history of each class began in the fall when the "freshies" entered the college "with smiles on their faces and hope in their hearts," only to face the inevitable confrontation with "sophs," whose constant hazing led finally to their coalescing in unity to establish a class identity. Students placed a high premium on class loyalty and esprit de corps. Thus, competition among the classes frequently turned into an all-consuming pastime, resulting in bloodied noses, black eyes, and the promise of a grudge match. Hazing carried into the college halls and occasionally into the class and dissection rooms where, to the consternation of faculty, pranks seemed to take precedence over studies. Freshmen were forced to occupy the rear seats of the amphitheater, wear their hair "just so long," bow and scrape before any sophomore, and "carry an absolutely unprofessional and inexperienced countenance."[31] The class of 1916 was set upon during one lecture period and painted in iodine.[32] All of this was intended, by custom, to forge class spirit. Of course, much of the hazing was settled during the annual rush of the fraternities and on the playing field (better known as the "field of honor") where classes challenged each other to football or other contact sports.

Battles to capture class flags were as common as Monday morning hangovers, and while Cincinnati newspapers made frequent reference to these antics, faculty seemed to fret only when they spilled into the street. One incident involved the effort by the class of 1911 to capture the sophomore flag, which flew from the cupola of the college building and which class members defended with clubs, red paint, rope, and muscle. Inspired by assurances of victory and having steeled themselves with sufficient beer to accomplish the task, the freshmen rushed to the top of an adjoining building and attempted to cross over to the institute and scale the cupola from an improvised ladder. Failing in their endeavor, they then filled squirt guns with ammonia water and charged the sophomore ranks, aiming at their eyes. This tactic succeeded, and, having replaced the sophomore flag with their own, the victors proceeded to march the defeated sophomores to Fountain Square where they "washed" them in public. Only then did the Cincinnati police intervene and bring the episode to an end. With ties of loyalty thus forged, the freshmen looked forward to their sophomore year and the opportunity to induct the next class of freshies into the college. "How blissful and sensational were those days!" recalled one student. "With the honors of the Class . . . at stake, we were forced to show the Freshmen, emphatically, their places in college life."[33]

By junior year, students had rolled down their trousers and took to wearing black derby hats and plain coats, hose, and ties. Occupied with more scientific deliberations and aware of the seriousness of their chosen profession, the class acquired a work ethic and began to contemplate—both collectively and individually—the implications of their chosen profession. Still, there were evenings at "Toney's," where they drank beer and played cards; late-night discussions and pranks at Lackey's boarding house; theater parties at the Standard; lunches of graham crackers and coffee at "The Dairy"; last-minute purchases at the Cincinnati Medical Book Company on 905 Race Street; an evening of fun at the Central Bowling Alleys on West Seventh Street; drinking parties on Vine Street; and the inevitable list of romances and broken hearts.[34] There was also the occasional confrontation between the unknowing dean and an irate dog owner who discovered that students had secured his pet hound for the "good of science."[35]

Some incidents attracted the ire of faculty and administrators. In 1922, one student advertised in the *Cincinnati Times-Star* for a wife, "any woman between the ages of eighteen and thirty, white and of good stock," who could finance his two remaining years of college. "I am at the end of my rope," he was quoted as saying. "Ambition is too strong to permit me to drop my efforts for an education. I cannot let price intervene. I must complete my studies. There is no other way." In explaining his situation, the student revealed that his immediate family had stopped supporting him and his education had been assumed by an uncle who agreed to trade the cost of his last two years of medical education for marriage to his daughter. Preferring a woman not related to him, who might make a similar offer, he had chosen to go to the press.

Secretary John K. Scudder called the student into his office and asked if he realized the "outrageousness of his behavior." In taking his problem to the press, the student had made an "exhibition of bad taste," which the faculty and trustees did not appreciate. Some even called for the student's expulsion. According to Scudder, the young man had said nothing to college authorities concerning his financial situation, having paid his fees just as other students. Although despondent because the faculty accused him of disgracing his alma mater, he reported that at least one young woman from Kentucky had responded to his offer.[36]

Student humor was no different from that at most schools. Faculty members were mocked for their most typical classroom comments. Lyman Watkins, whose classes were dull, seemed always to be saying, "Wake up, Doctor; wake up!" and Edwin R. Freeman, who was a stickler for protocol, saying, "I'll not proceed until you take your feet down." The largest "live-stock owner" among the students was the one who owned the largest collection of "ponies." The class remembered Dr. B. M. Alleman for his lecture on contraceptives; Doc Andress for his political digressions; Dean Byron H. Nellans for his enthusiasm; Dr. J. M. Haynes for his eccentricities; Miss Lennon, who "bossed" the clinic; and the first visit to Cincinnati General Hospital.[37]

Every class had its poets who were held in high esteem by comrades. The following verse refers to the students' reliance on "ponies" to get them through their courses.

> To Horse! To Horse!
> O Shades of Polyphase, so darkly known,
> Curse of a hundred toiling Studes.
> Beneath its awful load we sweat and groan,
> Pursuing bugs and germs and other bosh.
> "Horse of a hundred rides, be with us yet—
> Lest we forget, lest we forget!"
>
> Oh Lab tests are a thing we all despise,
> For neither rhyme nor reason there avail.
> 'Tis sickening to comprehend, the size
> Of tests that in that place prevail.
> "So horse of a hundred rides, be with us yet—
> Lest we forget, lest we forget!"[38]

School colors were burnt-orange and black, and each class chose its own colors, flower, and motto. The 1911 graduating class's colors were red and white, the flower the American beauty, the motto "Inest sua gratia parvis," and the class yell

> Macertate 'em; Percolate 'em; Rah! Rah! Rah!
> Sterilize 'em; Immunize 'em; Wah! Wah! Wah!
> Amputation, Medication,
> Way to Health (or Heaven)
> Anything, Any Style.
> Nineteen-eleven.[39]

By contrast, the class of 1912 had colors of red and black, a red rose, a motto of "Move on to better Things," and the yell

Hull—a—ba—lo, Hul—a—ba—loo.
Nineteen-twelve
Zim—Zam—Zoo![40]

The class of 1913 had a similarly festive yell—

Hawkeye, Hawkeye, Buckeye, Buzz.
Wuz I an Eclectic? Well I guess I wuz.
Hobble gobble! Razzle dazzle,
Sis—Boom—Bah.
Nineteen-thirteen, Rah! Rah! Rah![41]

Students wrote and sang songs prepared by their classmen. One popular song, written by J. Garfield Smalley of the class of 1916, was sung at commencements and other notable events involving alumni.

College Song
O Father Eclectic, our voices we'll raise
And sound in thy honor our anthems of praise
From Wooster (Beach) to Scudder our hearts beat with pride
And loyal thy children who stand by thy side.

Chorus
All hail then hail to the orange and the black
While sickness reigns and Doctors replace quacks
We are loyal and true to our Eclectic School,
Are loyal and true to our Eclectic School.

From waif by the wayside to wealth on the hill
They call us to visit, we never stand still
In love do we render the ministering hand
Our motto as students "to help all we can."

Eclectic, we promise when far from thy breast
To follow thy guidance and heed thy behest
Our aim and our honor to relieve the distressed
From these this great blessing, forgetful the rest.[42]

Yet another popular song was "Our College," words and music by C. S. Palmer, class of 1917.

Our College
Eclectic old, to thee our praise we sing,
To thee all love and honor we will bring;
Thy fame of other days, thy gifts so free,
Call us today, to sing our praise to thee.

Chorus
Love and honor to Eclectic our college old and grand
Proudly we shall ever hail they over all the land,
Alma Mater, now we praise thee, our song shall ever be,
Love and honor to Eclectic our dear old E.M.C.

Thy halls, thy lecture-rooms to us so dear,
The bum-room that the students filled with cheer,
The dear old bell that called us to our place,
Are memories fond, that time can ne'er efface.

Thy teachings we believe and will obey,
On land, on sea, wherever we may stray,
Our duty ever in our loyalty,
To guard thy name through all eternity.[43]

FRATERNITIES AND CLUB SPORTS

Fraternity life at EMI differed little from colleges in Cincinnati or elsewhere. The first fraternity dedicated to the principles of eclecticism was the Alpha chapter of Tau Epsilon, founded at the college in 1896 and chartered in 1901. Several years later, chapters of Tau Epsilon were established at eclectic colleges in Kansas City, Missouri; Lincoln, Nebraska; and Atlanta, Georgia. The fraternity closed at the time of the school's reorganization in 1929 but opened again in 1934.[44] Theta Epsilon, organized in November 1935, held its first "smoker" a month later in the Hotel Sinton to acquaint undergraduates with the purposes and ideals of the fraternity. It also organized pledge dances at the Kemper Lane Hotel, interfraternity dances at the Cincinnati Club, and public discussions at the college on topics of interest in medicine.[45]

The EMI Club, representing a coalition of fraternity and nonfraternity men, organized as Sigma Theta in protest against the existing stereotype of hell-raising fraternities. Although intending to affiliate with a national fraternity, it abandoned the idea and, instead, received a charter from the state of Ohio in 1907. It was the first of the fraternal orders to reorganize in 1934. Dedicated to liberty, research, and fraternity, Sigma Theta had the reputation of being more highbrow than the other organizations at the college.[46]

The Aesculapians, comprising yet another fraternal organization, took root in December 1933 when a group of sophomores drew up a constitution and submitted it to Dean Nellans for approval. Its purpose was "to foster a spirit of cooperation in medical affairs both in undergraduate as well as in graduate life; to advance the principles of Eclecticism, and to uphold the ethics of the medical profession." During regular meetings of the society, students read or delivered talks, the subjects of which were usually taken from the "borderlines" of medicine where new advances were not yet included in textbooks or in classroom lectures. Through these discussions, students had the opportunity to hear new ideas and gain experience delivering a paper to the group. Though not technically a fraternity, the society fostered a spirit of fraternalism and cooperation among its members.[47]

Fraternities competed for students and encouraged a wholesome rivalry. Each year began with class elections, which included any number of fraternity intrigues, followed by a rush season when the competition for new members was most spirited. At the close of rush, each fraternity hosted a banquet for its new members. Thereafter classes settled in for the academic year—except for rivalries that existed for the hospital internships and other class honors.[48]

The local YMCA was a favorite of many students unable or unwilling to pay fraternity dues. Students frequently used its gymnasium, baths, parlors, and reading rooms. Its members set aside one hour each week to assemble for a short service of song and prayer, followed by an address of a minister from one of the Cincinnati churches, a missionary worker, or a member of the faculty.[49]

Like other colleges, EMC offered its students opportunities to participate in team sports, including football and baseball. The members of the football team wore black sweaters with the letter *E* blazoned in orange on the front, while the basketball team members wore orange sweaters over black crewnecks. Their competition was local

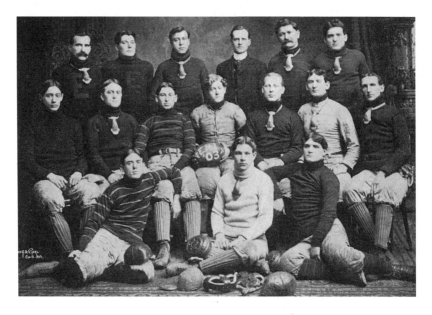

The EMI football team, 1903. Courtesy of the Lloyd Library and Museum.

and included Xavier, Ohio Dental College, Cincinnati Law School, YMCA Law School, Lane Seminary, Woodward, Lawrenceburg, and the School of Commerce.[50]

Student Theses

Theses written in the last year of studies were a vital part of the medical student's preparation. Ranging from ten to forty pages in length, they reflected the concerns of the time. In the 1840s and 1850s, students felt the pulse of reform much more acutely. D. H. Morgan's thesis in 1846 read remarkably like the American Declaration of Independence, beginning with the words: "When in the course of human events it becomes necessary for the student to comply with the requisitions of an institution by presenting them for consideration of his professors some production from his pen." Morgan then explained his reasons for leaving the established path of regular medicine to "join with those who have deemed it conducive to the best interests of mankind that a reformation in that science should be affected."

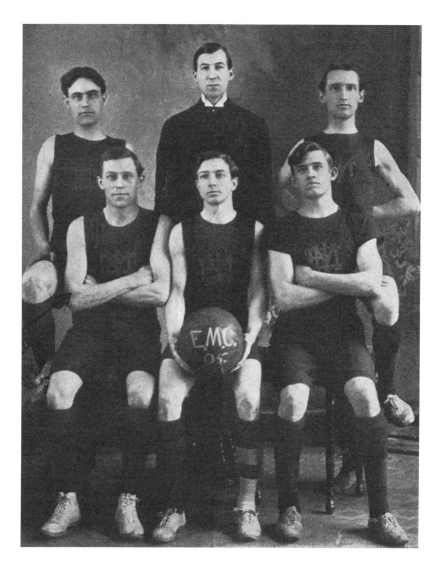

The EMI basketball team, 1904–5. Courtesy of the Lloyd Library and Museum.

It should be the great object of all classes and associations of men to offer the greatest possible good with the least evil to their fellow man and I hold these truths self evident that whenever the means become destructive of the end they were assigned to accomplish it is the right nay the imperative duty of such as discover the error to alter or abolish it and to institute the necessary changes and establish such principles and organize its power in such form as shall seem most likely to effect the safety and happiness of mankind. Such has been the case in medical science. While the practitioners were enjoying the confidence of community honoured with seats in high places and rolling in wealth and splendour liberally furnished by their deluded patrons their great object seemed to be to shroud in darkness and mystery the healing art (falsely so called) and introduce from time to time remedies called in almost every instance from a kingdom which professes no life giving principle and whose particles cannot be assimilated with the human system.[51]

Morgan went on to complain that allopathy consisted of men who, when called upon to cure, provided little more than silence for discretion, a "vacant stare" for wisdom, and a regular license for manslaughter.[52] These pretenders had succeeded in making credulous followers believe there was only one authentic group of physicians while castigating medical reformers as little more than "steam and pepper doctors." Morgan insisted that a clear distinction existed between the medical reform movement and the "deluded followers" of Samuel Thomson who had formulated "a heterogeneous map of absurdities . . . dependent upon indolence and cupidity for its origin and . . . support." He judged Thomson incapable of formulating a rational system of practice and too lazy to have qualified himself for it after the fact. His was a "vaporous science" built on the "grossest errors" of empiricism.[53]

In the class of 1848, Charles C. Crandall of Birmingham, Ohio, submitted a thesis "On the Responsibilities and Duties of a Physician." Eleven pages long, it amounted to little more than a letter home discussing the need for the young practitioner to maintain a "scrutinizing eye" as he attended to his practice; to conduct himself with comportment and respect for the healing art; to avoid the "abominable practice" of prescribing calomel and antimony; to adhere to principles instead of shifting "with each breath of public opinion"; to attend the wants of the poor; to know the integrity of the person filling his prescriptions; and to keep concise notes on all patients to compile medical statistics.[54]

Student Nathan L. Van Zandt of Cincinnati argued that medicine acted by way of a "dynamic force peculiar to itself, and capable of exerting its own . . . special influence upon the organism." Enamored as much by homeopathy as by Joseph Rodes Buchanan's views on phrenology and psychometrics, he wrote in his 1850 thesis of impressible individuals who could obtain the full physiological effects from certain medicines merely by holding them in their hand. All medicines, he reasoned, acted in a similar manner—that is, had an affinity for a specific organ or a stimulating effect upon the seat of nervous power in the brain. The physician could cure disease "upon philosophical principles with a certainty unknown to the present notion and empirical practice of medicine." Van Zandt explained that, although similar in theory to homeopathy, the eclectics had carried these principles further and that this was the most formidable contribution of the reformed school to the healing art.[55]

Not surprisingly, student theses reflected the same ideological pursuits that consumed the faculty at EMI: frequent reference to intellectual freedom; opposition to the exclusiveness of allopathic theory; numerous references to the horrors of calomel, antimony, and the lancet; and the importance of being identified as "reformers in principle and practice." Student theses exuded optimism in the ultimate direction of medical reform and adherence to the natural (Christian) duties of physicians. Two areas of particular interest were hydropathy (using a combination of frequent bathing and simple remedies) and electricity. Both students and faculty viewed them as safe and supportive of the body's vital system. Although students identified prominent allopathic doctors whose therapeutical techniques had proven useful, they found little to admire in allopathy as a system. It was, wrote one student, the "most foul and corrupt system of Practice that has prevailed for centuries, ten times worse than any Experience that ever visited the face of the globe."[56]

Student theses were almost chiliastic in their view of the future. A new era was dawning upon the world and the "old order of things fast passing away," observed M. H. Siegmund Saches in his 1852 thesis.

Monopolies, oppression, and injustice of all kinds were "tottering on their last legs" because of the power of popular opinion. The structure of religion and government was changing and, with it, social life, arts, and sciences were assuming "a new character and new relations." The same was also true of the privileged and all who had "encroached upon the sacred rights of others." And in the midst of these changes, a new age of medicine was emerging along with a new class of medical reformers to replace "old Dr. Calomel."[57] Saches urged his fellow students to keep eclecticism before the people and to convince Dr. Calomel and his disciples to lay aside their prejudices and join the cause. Unlike other sectarians, the eclectics held up to the world no single leader. Samuel Hahnemann, Vincenz Priessnitz, Anton Mesmer, and Samuel Thomson were great men in their own way, but the eclectic school had freed itself from the iconoclasm of a single leader and a single theory and practice.[58]

The eclectics had but a few restrictions to their liberality. The first was the exclusion of most minerals from their materia medica believing that, "having no affinity for the elements of the body, [they] can only . . . act as foreign substances and consequently as continual irritants on some or all parts of the organism, creating an artificial disease, that is frequently found more intractable, than the original disease." The second principle was to employ plants that were indigenous to the United States. Believing that providence had provided a remedy for every disease, and that disease and remedy "will generally be found at no great distance from one another," the eclectics held forth that American doctors would eventually discover a sufficient number of indigenous plants to replace imported ones.[59]

Any number of theses heralded the strengths and peculiarities of eclectic practice and reserved for Old School doctors the shibboleth of "hunkers" for their obsolete regimens. No theses involved original research and few, if any, provided a review of the literature. Most did little more than restate in general terms the conclusions and prejudices of the faculty.

GRADUATING CLASSES

The graduating class of 1911 published the school's first yearbook. Titled *The Skull—1911*, and dedicated to secretary John K. Scudder, it promised to "praise indiscriminately and to criticize consistently." The book contained pictures of each member of the graduating class and a short resume that included the individual's place of origin, high school and college preparatory work, club sport and fraternity, nickname ("Ozone," "Osler," "Deacon," "The Tincture"), and a brief statement to memorialize the student's presence.[60]

Commencements were held in the Scottish Rite Cathedral at 417 Broadway or in Memorial Hall at Elm and Grant Streets. During the years of John M. Scudder's leadership, they consisted of a march, followed by benediction and music, and punctuated by a "Report of the Session" by Scudder, a "Valedictory Address" by one of the graduates, and an "Address" by a member of the faculty.[61] Later commencement exercises were more lively events beginning with an invocation and followed by music (such as "Orange Blossoms" by Victor Herbert), the "Dean's Report," more music, the conferring of degrees, music, an address, more music, and the benediction. In the May 20, 1929, commencement exercise, Jake Bohrer's orchestra provided a sampling of popular melodies of the day.[62]

Graduates were also invited to a luncheon at the Business Man's Club in Cincinnati as guests of the William S. Merrell Company. This followed a tour of the company's laboratory at Fifth and Pike Streets, intended to acquaint graduates with the quality of the company's medicines and hopefully build a strong relationship with the young doctors in future years. Secretary John K. Scudder, Rolla L. Thomas, and Byron Nellans usually accompanied the graduates on these site visits.[63]

The Alumni

The first alumni association for the college, organized in 1846, became dormant shortly before the Civil War and reorganized following the fire that nearly destroyed the college in 1869. During the dedication of the college's new addition in 1871, the association announced its officers and promised to become an important force in the school's future.[64] Because of the proprietary nature of the college, however, the alumni association played only a secondary role in its activities. Symptomatic of this, meetings were held irregularly until 1890 when new energy among the membership resulted in a more organized and aggressive approach. The causes for the alumni's renewed activity were increased interest in the changing nature of medical education and licensing and the realization that the future status of eclecticism

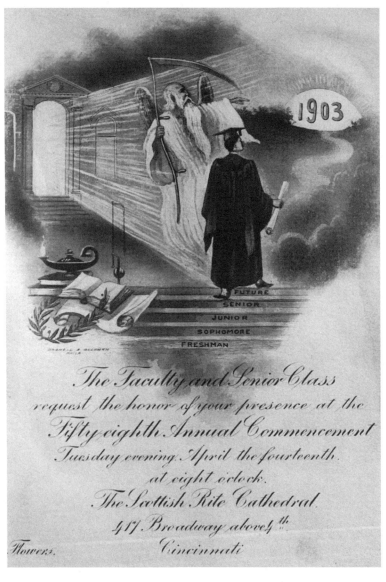

Commencement invitation, 1903. Courtesy of the Lloyd Library and Museum.

depended as much upon the success and continuation of the institute as it did upon the success of its alumni. To ensure this, the association turned to the school's graduates for endowment monies to support the college.[65]

Typically, the alumni association met during the week of commencement in the lower lecture hall in the institute at 630 West Sixth Street. The format for the meeting remained the same from one year to the next: a treasurer's report, update on the endowment, valedictory address to the new graduating class, president's address, a roll call of past graduates in attendance, induction of the new graduating class into the association, and a report on new projects, followed by the election of new officers.[66]

In 1909, the charter of the institute was amended by a general act of the Ohio legislature that enabled any educational institution chartered prior to the state constitution of 1851 to cancel its stock and turn the school's management over to a self-perpetuating board of trustees. Among the beneficiaries of this legislation, faculty at EMI and other private colleges were eligible to arrange teachers' pensions through the Carnegie Foundation. EMI availed itself of the legislation not only to change its charter, thereby helping the faculty, but chose the opportunity to eliminate the word "institute" from its official name, which, along with "academy" and "seminary," had grown into disuse.[67] Under new operating papers, a board of trustees was created consisting of not less than eleven or more than fifteen members chosen for three-year terms, five of whom had to be graduates of the college.[68] Having obtained through the reorganization a greater share in the decision making of the college, the alumni hoped that "the day is not far distant when our laboratories and chairs of didactic teaching shall be endowed, and grounds and buildings added to meet increasing requirements."[69]

By 1911, there were more than four thousand graduates of the college, of whom over 1,800 were still engaged in practice. Of that number, 450 were members of the alumni association paying an annual fee of one dollar. According to alumni records, graduates of the institute practiced in every state and the island possessions of the United States and occupied positions in the army, navy, and on U.S. examining boards. Graduates also practiced in Europe and the British Isles and served as missionary doctors in India, China, Japan, Australia, Africa, New Zealand, and South America.[70]

CHAPTER FIVE

Presiding over Change

Deans Rolla L. Thomas (1904–31), Eben B. Shewman (1934–35), and Byron H. Nellans (1931–33, 1935–39) led the college through its final years of fundraising, reorganization, self-study, and closing. On their watch the college faced its greatest challenges and most bitter defeats. Like their predecessors, they continued to hire faculty from among the graduates of the college. In 1908, twenty of the twenty-five faculty were alumni; the oldest, Linus E. Russell, had graduated from EMI in 1872. Most, however, had graduated between 1881 and 1900. Twenty years later, the mix of faculty had changed only slightly. By then, thirty-two out of forty-three of the instructional staff were alumni, with William N. Mundy, who had graduated from EMI in 1883, the oldest. Hiring remained the responsibility of secretary John K. Scudder, who as the managing executive officer, set most school policies.

The first of the deans, Rolla L. Thomas (1857–1932) of 792 East McMillan Street, was a deeply committed Methodist, physically strong, and happiest when engaged in several different projects at a time. Thomas was born in 1857 in Harrison, Hamilton County, Ohio. His father, Milton L. Thomas, graduated from the Louisville Medical College in 1854 and the Eclectic Medical Institute in 1857 and served as preceptor to his son and, before him, to John Milton Scudder. Young Thomas eventually attended Indiana Asbury University (now DePauw University) in Greencastle, Indiana, graduating in 1878. That same year he matriculated at EMI and graduated in 1880. He then opened a practice in Harrison and remained there until 1887, when he was appointed adjunct professor of principles and practice of medicine and assumed the bulk of John M. Scudder's teaching duties during his final illness. Following Scudder's death, Thomas was appointed full

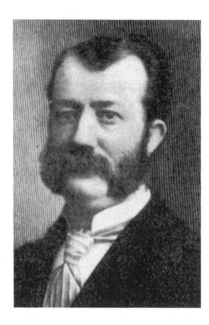

Rolla L. Thomas, M.D. (1857–1932), dean of EMC (1904–31). Courtesy of the Lloyd Library and Museum.

professor, lecturing once each week on the principles of medicine and three times a week on the practice of medicine. "His speech, his very looks, breathed a compassionate feeling for others," wrote eclectic historian Harvey Wickes Felter. Colleagues described him as fearless, upright, genial, sympathetic, and, above all, a Christian gentleman and physician; not surprisingly, he was often asked to give inspirational talks at the college chapter of the YMCA. In the classroom, Thomas tempered his lectures with moderation and, although strict in his quizzing, was considered a fair grader. When Dean Frederick Locke died in 1903, the trustees appointed Thomas, by then immensely popular among both students and faculty colleagues, as his replacement. Thomas also served that year as president of the National Eclectic Medical Association, which convened the largest body of eclectics ever gathered at the World's Fair in St. Louis. Besides his administrative duties, Thomas maintained a successful general and obstetrical practice, leaving the management of the college to John K. Scudder.[1]

The early days of Thomas's deanship coincided with some of the more momentous changes occurring in medical education. For one thing, older sectarianism no longer retained the credibility it once held in the public arena. Although sectarians still demonstrated many admirable traits, observed John B. Nichols in his presidential address before the Medical Society of the District of Columbia, they had "nothing to offer in the way of resources, methods or principles that regular medicine does not possess; and the continued existence of the eclectic sect seemed simply a perpetuation of a name and organization after the reasons that may have originally called it into being have ceased to operate."[2] Physio-medicalism had become moribund, its last college closing in 1911, and homeopathy seemed little more than an artifact of the Middle Ages when the smelling of a sugar pellet promised mysterious potency and cure. Actually, few of homeopathy's followers still employed its original doctrines, preferring instead to move closer to regular medicine.

The years of Thomas's deanship corresponded with intensified efforts to recruit new students, urging eclectics to forward the names of any interested students before the Ohio and New York boards raised their entrance requirements beyond the present high school standards.[3] The school's marketing efforts were similar to strategies underway at the 101 other medical colleges in the United States seeking to capitalize on their investments in new laboratories, buildings, better equipment, larger hospital facilities, and full-time salaried instructors. All were struggling in some manner to modernize. Many of these colleges were closing or merging because of increased pressures from the Council on Medical Education and the Association of American Medical Colleges. Between 1906 and 1914, the number of regular medical colleges fell from 130 to eighty-seven, with a 35.4 percent decline in graduates. For homeopathic schools, there was a corresponding decline from twenty-two to ten schools, with 63.3 percent fewer graduates. For the eclectics, the figures were even more ominous. From a high of ten schools in 1901 to four in 1914, eclectics showed a decrease of 68.3 percent in the number of graduates.[4]

ALUMNAL EFFORTS

The 1911 meeting of the Alumnal Association noted the college's new building at 630 West Sixth Street adjacent to Seton Hospital on the west. The land, equipment, and furniture were valued at $55,500 and mortgaged for $15,000. Recognizing that the college received no revenue from public taxation and that the running expenses of the college and bond fees were paid entirely from tuition and endowment, the association well understood the demands on its members' collective pocketbook.[5] In addition to fund-raising activities, the association inaugurated "Clinic Week" for the benefit of the alumni— a form of continuing education consisting of free lectures and clinical demonstrations at the college and at Seton Hospital during commencement week.[6]

The next year, the association sent out a circular letter to nearly two thousand alumni reporting on the college and the upcoming commencement exercises. The association asked each graduate to pledge ten dollars per year toward the purchase of laboratory equipment and to support salaried instructors. In addition, the association authorized a marble tablet for the vestibule of the college commemorating the professors who had taught from 1845 to 1875. By 1913, pledges to the permanent endowment fund amounted to $30,343.[7]

In 1916, the Alumnal Association sent out fourteen hundred invitations to graduates who were nonmembers, asking them to attend the forthcoming Clinic Week and to consider joining the association. The invitation included information on the upcoming commencement exercises at Memorial Hall and described the participation of the junior class in the 320-bed Tuberculosis Hospital as well as the clinical opportunities available at the Seton Hospital Clinics. The association proudly mentioned that EMC was one of sixty-two medical colleges recognized by the Ohio State Medical Board, one of sixty-one accredited for examination and reciprocity in Pennsylvania, and one of sixty-nine colleges registered by the New York regents.[8]

Four years later, Thomas and Scudder sent out another letter to friends and alumni. They referred to the college's recent bulletins, which listed the class year and mailing address of each living graduate and a brief history of the college prepared by Harvey Wickes Felter. They noted that of every one hundred matriculants, thirty-five resulted from the recruiting efforts of the college, thirty came as transfers from other schools, and only thirty-five were there through the efforts of alumni and other eclectics. Believing that more students should come through the recruiting efforts of alumni, the dean and secretary encouraged eclectics to speak before their local high schools, urging interested young men and women to attend Earlham, Miami of Ohio, or other nearby colleges for a premedical course of study before matriculating at EMC. The two men were equally concerned that graduates and alumni donate annually to the endowment fund of the college. "Your college is rated 'B' by the AMA," they explained. "If you want it placed in 'Class A,' you must help us increase our Endowment Fund to a Half Million Dollars, which will then produce an additional income of $25,000 per year." Even with a B rating, Thomas and Scudder assured alumni that the college continued to have a "good reputation" and was fully recognized in forty-three states.[9]

By 1923, the endowment had reached $60,000, but not enough to sustain the school's growing needs. Association officers reminded alumni that the demands of state boards and the AMA's Council on Medical Education required the employment of at least six paid instructors who worked full-time at the college—a criterion that the school would ultimately fail to achieve.[10]

Ironically, the building that the college had so proudly erected in 1910 proved woefully inadequate for the needs of modern medicine. Designed for didactic instruction, it lacked sufficient laboratory and research space for students and faculty. Moreover, as much as the college enjoyed its proximity to and relationship with Seton Hospital, the facilities were too small to sustain the level of clinical activity needed for the junior and senior years. There were too few beds, and the hospital failed to provide sufficient number and variety of experiences.

NEW BUILDING SCHEME

In 1923, John Uri Lloyd and his brother Nelson Ashley Lloyd informed the trustees that they had purchased land at the southwest corner of June Street and Essex Place, across from Bethesda Hospital, for a new college building.[11] Thomas and Scudder responded enthusiastically to the offer, promising to lay the proposal before the National Eclectic Medical Association at its next annual meeting. They established a building and endowment fund and estimated the amount needed to bring the school a class-A rating at $1,250,000, which included construction of a new college adjoining Bethesda Hospital, a full complement of equipment, scholarships, full-time salaried faculty, and a healthy endowment.[12] Caught up in the enthusiasm, John Uri promised to equip the college with a botanical research laboratory. Hopes were high as the campaign got underway.[13]

A year later, the building and endowment fund committee reported a total of $158,902 pledged; $58,170 paid; and $18,500 collected in life policies.[14] Within two years, the college had acquired 175 life policies for $196,000, with an additional $300,000 pending.[15] The largest single gift, aside from the land, came from the Lloyd brothers in the amount of $8,575 each, and the largest life policy came from Dr. Joseph A. Munk of Los Angeles, an 1863 graduate of the college. Most other gifts, including life policies, were for much smaller amounts.[16]

Following an initial flurry of pledges and supportive articles in Cincinnati and other regional newspapers, the campaign faltered, with most commitments made in the form of insurance policies. The funds needed to sustain the college beyond the construction of the new building, and the dollars required to support full-time salaried instructors, clinical facilities, and modern equipment simply did not materialize. Loyalty to the college, the trustees learned, was skin deep. By the end of 1925, two years into the campaign, the trustees reluctantly concluded that the prospect of a new college building appeared unlikely.[17]

Discouraged by the inability to raise funds and realizing, too, that the college lacked monies beyond tuition to support ongoing needs, the trustees ordered Dean Thomas to halt matriculation of the freshman class in 1926. While instruction of students in the three upper classes would continue through graduation, the trustees concluded, albeit reluctantly, that unless the college could operate at a level commensurate with other medical colleges and in step with the curricular and fiscal parameters suggested by the AMA's Council on Medical Education, they had no recourse but to close. They then decided to postpone a formal vote to end the charter but agreed that, unless the school's financial condition improved, permanent closure would come with the graduation of the last class.[18]

In August 1928, the officers of the Alumnal Association called for a special meeting in response to two letters. The first, written by Byron H. Nellans, reminded the alumni and friends of the college that the future of eclecticism was in jeopardy and that "factions, petty jealousies [and] discordant notes must be abolished" before its future could be assured. This required harmony among members and an end to the secrecy surrounding the management of the college. Above all else, the Alumnal Association must become an active and integral player in the college's future. Its role included participation in the selection of the college's trustees; a more active involvement in the work of the building and endowment committee; supporting the hiring of a new executive secretary; taking greater fiscal responsibility for clinical and hospital needs; and supporting the local, state, and national needs of eclectics. This latter challenge included meeting the requirements of the American Medical Association; testing the legal rights of eclecticism; and building the endowment through appeals to drug manufacturers, alumni, women's auxiliaries, and other potential benefactors. Finally, Nellans urged more regular meetings of the association; raising the annual fees; publishing the association's activities; and proving to the AMA that eclecticism would not waiver in its commitment to modernize its facilities and adhere to the cause of reform. "Hold sacred to our trust and do not waiver in our cause," Nellans argued. "Now is the time to act."[19]

The appeal was followed by a second letter to the alumni by W. N. Mundy, president of the association. In it, he wrote: "The time for action has arrived. Already there has been too much procrastination!" He encouraged those supporting their alma mater to meet on August 1 at the Gibson Hotel in Cincinnati. Mundy challenged the alumni by telling them that the change in the college's charter in 1909 had made it the property of the alumni. Unfortunately, "we have taken practically no interest in it. NO COLLEGE has ever succeeded that had not the GOOD WILL and moral influence of its Alumni." Whether the school continued or not depended ultimately upon the solution agreed upon at the meeting. "There comes a crisis in the life of every man and institution," Mundy observed, "and OURS IS HERE. Will we successfully pass through the crisis? IT IS FOR YOU TO ANSWER."[20]

One hundred alumni responded to his appeal by attending the special August meeting. After intense debate, the members appointed a liaison committee charged with the task of improving communication between the association and the trustees of the college and exploring the hiring of a new executive officer. The members also recommended republishing the college bulletin, which had been discontinued, and developing a plan to raise the school's endowment, thereby satisfying the funding needs for a class-A institution. Members also urged the college to solicit donations from philanthropic individuals and organizations outside eclecticism, specifically the National Grange and industrialist Henry Ford.[21]

As early as 1925, the National Grange had expressed alarm at the growing shortage of country doctors. In 1906, approximately 33,000 physicians served communities of one thousand or less. By 1924, only 27,000 physicians continued to serve this same population, and Grange investigations indicated that almost a third of the towns that had physicians in 1914 had none in 1925. Equally troublesome, the average age of the rural doctor in the study was fifty-two years, while the average age at death of American physicians was sixty-two. Thus, the Grange predicted, the present generation of rural doctors would perish in ten years. Worse yet, smaller and smaller percentages of recently graduated doctors chose to practice in rural districts. Troubled by this ominous information, the Grange appealed to the American Medical Association to produce more general practitioners. "The family doctor is rapidly becoming extinct," it warned in its statement to the AMA. "He is being supplemented by the specialist to a degree not warranted under practical conditions. If the supply of country doctors is to be replenished, these doctors must come from among the young men and women of the country districts, as was the case in former times." Grange officers observed that only in rare instances could "the son of a farmer hope to enter the medical profession owing to the expense of his education." While not advocating the lowering of standards, the association urged a more practical education that required less time and less specialization and that gave greater deference to patient care than to the laboratory sciences.[22]

The eclectics were buoyed by the Grange's appeal to the American Medical Association but felt that the farm organization had directed its appeal to the wrong group of doctors. C. W. Beaman, M.D., president of the National Eclectic Medical Association, reported that medical education had become too lengthy a process. By the time students had completed their studies in the urban areas where most medical colleges were now located, few had any inclination to set up their practices in rural communities. "Specialization emphasized during [their] college courses, causes [them] to adopt some of the many departments of medicine . . . and to think little of general medicine, which is the background of the family physician or the country doctor," Beaman remarked. The Grange, he said, advocated a different method of training, requiring less time and less specialization and with modified entrance requirements, to permit a "country boy" to study medicine and then return to his rural environment. However, this was impossible under the "radical changes in standards now in vogue," he said. The health needs of rural America could not be solved simply by transporting every patient twenty-five to a hundred miles by car or train to the nearest urban hospital.[23]

The fifty-eighth-annual National Eclectic Medical Association met in Lexington, Kentucky, on June 19–22, 1928, and focused much of its activity on the issues raised by the Grange. C. W. Beaman opened the meeting by announcing that the eclectics were interested in returning medicine to the general practitioner. "Most [regular] schools have been dominated by the specialist in surgery and its allied branches and this being more spectacular has interested the student more deeply than general medicine," he remarked to the nearly one thousand assembled delegates. "The wane of the family physician and the advent of the young specialist are robbing medicine of the carefully equipped bedside practitioner."[24] In an age of specialists, the eclectics hoped for a revival of the "old-fashioned family doctor who would sit again by the bedside of the sick child." With the advent of the young specialist, medicine had had been robbed of its most respected element, a loss felt more deeply in rural America.[25]

"The greatest call of humanity today is for the general practitioner, the good old family doctor," remarked Nellans to the opening session. "The family physician with the traditions which are so honestly his by dent of service to humanity is certainly needed today," he reminded the gathering. "We have always contended that the real purpose of the medical college was to graduate men for general practice. . . . The man desiring to specialize should do so after he has practiced general medicine for a number of years, acquainted himself with general disease conditions, and found himself so that he knows to what field he is especially adapted."[26]

This wishful thinking was a frequent topic of discussion among older faculty and alumni at EMI but less so among younger doctors who had accepted the consequences of curricular reform. For this latter group, the issue was not specialism versus the values of the family practitioner; it was whether the eclectics were genuinely committed to educational reform. The difference was real and represented a distinction between the empiricism of the laboratory—the power of observation and the inductive method of scientific study—and an older didactism.

Hoping to keep the Alumnal Association focused on the needs of the college, Mundy called for another special meeting in November 1928. "As has so often been said," he wrote, "a school is what its alumni make it. Point, if you can, to any school, save only state or municipal universities that have succeeded, whose success did not depend upon the good will and gifts of its alumni." Clearly the die had been cast. The college, whose record and whose existence had been cherished by its graduates for more than eighty years, was in mortal danger because of the demands made upon all medical schools by state licensing boards, the AMA, foundations, and discipline-based societies.[27]

High expectations notwithstanding, only thirty-five alumni attended the November meeting. Hoping to augment membership by including graduates from extinct eclectic colleges who were now little more than "medical orphans," Mundy encouraged the association members to accept graduates from those "reputable but defunct institutions, providing they are legal practitioners of medicine, and in good repute." If they contributed money, they could even vote on issues involving the college.[28] Mundy also assured the small gathering that the trustees welcomed the work done by the association and had even requested nominations for membership to the board. But, aside from these two actions, the meeting lacked the enthusiasm that had sparked the earlier August convention. If anything, it signaled that the responsibility for the college's future would continue to be carried on the shoulders of the faculty and administration rather than by alumni. In short, the Alumnal Association lacked in both numbers and commitment to fulfill the promises associated with the reorganization of the college charter. On paper, the college operated on behalf of the association. In fact, the college remained in the hands of a few caring and committed individuals—but hands too few and too frail to ensure its future.

In May 1929, C. S. Amidon, M.D., chairman of the Alumnal Association, informed the trustees that the AMA's Council on Medical Education continued to push for medical school curriculum reform nationally. This meant for EMC the hiring of full-time instructors, maintaining properly equipped laboratories, and raising a minimum of $25,000 annually over and above student fees. The assets of the col-

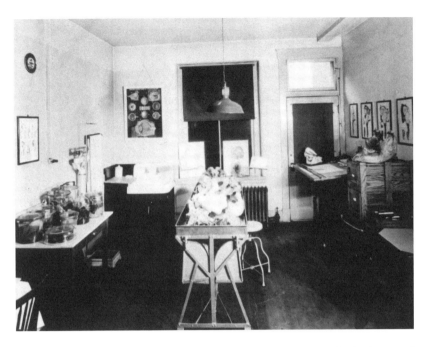

Department of Anatomy preparation room, 1930. Courtesy of the Lloyd Library and Museum.

lege included a building and equipment valued about $130,000; donated property upon which to build a new college; approximately $200,000 in insurance payable to the college and earning $2,500 annually in dividends; and a "long and honorable career" with an "honest desire to teach medicine in accordance with present-day requirements." On the deficit side, Amidon sensed that the alumni felt handicapped in supporting the college because of their lack of power within the broader medical community and an imperfect understanding of the requirements of present-day medical education. These impediments, he explained, translated into a lack of money and influence to help the college in its hour of need.[29]

At the same May meeting, the trustees also learned of a conversation between Dr. N. P. Colwell, first secretary to the Council on Medical Education, and a committee consisting of C. S. Amidon, Judge John Weld Peck, Charles W. Beaman, and Byron H. Nellans. The purpose of the meeting was to obtain an informal, but honest, assessment

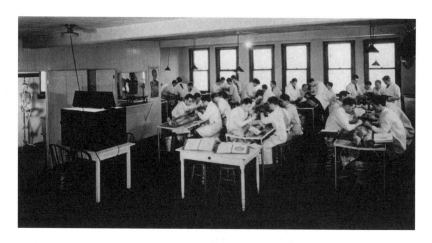

Anatomy laboratory, 1930. Courtesy of the Lloyd Library and Museum.

of the condition of the college and an opinion as to whether the college could receive a class-A rating if it reopened. In his most diplomatic language, Colwell explained that while he was personally satisfied that the college might eventually establish a proper hospital affiliation, hire an acceptable teaching faculty, and secure the funding necessary to ensure permanency, he could not vouch for the opinion of the other council members. On hearing Colwell's less-than-enthusiastic response, the committee concluded that the school's future was "hopeless," its greatest handicap being a proper hospital affiliation. Judge Peck reasoned that the college had five options: first, make a successful fund drive that would result in a new teaching college and sufficient endowment monies to maintain it; second, continue as a school "of limited field" that would severely restrict graduates and make it "an outcast medical school"; third, become a postgraduate training site unaffiliated with the Council on Medical Education, perpetuating the "useful principles" of eclectic medicine; fourth, seek an affiliation with another Ohio university, relinquishing the name of the school but hopefully retaining a chair in eclectic medicine; or fifth, closing permanently.[30]

In response to Peck's options, the board held a special meeting two months later to discuss the overall condition of the college and its prospects for continuing. After much anguished discussion, the trustees voted to close the college "at the earliest moment" and dismiss the employees as soon as their services could be dispensed with. At the same time, the trustees appointed a search committee to hire a qualified business manager to continue the quest for development funds. With no new matriculants and the graduation of the last class in May 1929, the AMA listed the school as "extinct," but the trustees asserted that the college was merely "resting" until a new building or a better solution materialized.[31]

With its closing, the college faced the immediate task of returning all insurance policies. The executive committee solved this dilemma by informing policy holders that they could either request a return of their polices or, preferably, substitute a cash pledge for the building campaign. The committee also considered an idea put forth by John Uri that, in the event the building campaign failed, a research center or laboratory be established to disseminate "authoritive" information relative to the principles of eclectic medicine. If done, the college could revert to "institute" status and, although it could grant no degrees, would remain free of interference from the Council on Medical Education and its parent institution, the American Medical Association.[32] The trustees accepted the proposal, but it was clear from their discussions that they had not given up hope of eventually reopening the college.[33]

On August 12, 1930, the trustees met again in a special meeting, this time in response to the sudden death of John K. Scudder. After passing appropriate resolutions of condolence to his family, the board appointed Charles W. Beaman to fill his unexpired term as treasurer. Rolla Thomas continued as dean of the faculty, Beaman served as both treasurer and secretary to the board, and Byron Nellans became assistant secretary and treasurer.[34]

Because of continuing low turnout at their meetings, the Alumnal Association decided to meet jointly with the annual gathering of national and state eclectic associations. In making this change, the association hoped to use these occasions to entice graduates of extinct schools to help support the only remaining eclectic college. The next several meetings of the association were uneventful except that attendance continued to drop. At the national convention in Little Rock, Arkansas, Secretary C. R. Campbell called the members to order since no other officer was present. The meeting ended abruptly after the secretary accepted a donation of three hundred dollars to the college and appealed to delinquent members to pay their dues. The results of the association's drive to boost membership proved to be so disappointing (the association admitted only three new members) that it authorized hiring a consultant to determine whether the college should matriculate a new class or remain closed.[35]

Responding to the association's recommendation, and concerned that the school might not be able to manage a successful fund-raising drive, Beaman and Nellans hired the consulting firm of Ketchum, Inc., of Pittsburgh to assess the college's potential. The report, which they shared with the board on March 28, 1931, "brought to light nothing new so far as methods of raising funds." The board accepted the report but refused to act on its implied recommendation and refused to end any hope of resurrecting the college. Instead, it decided to push ahead "to rehabilitate the institution, independent of any dictation" from the AMA.[36]

At the annual meeting of the National Eclectic Medical Association in Indianapolis, June 16–19, 1931, delegates urged the trustees to reopen the college and appoint a full-time executive secretary to manage its affairs. The association, spurred by the jingoism of the delegates, challenged the college to operate exclusively as an eclectic institution, "entirely free from the domination or dictation" of the AMA's Council on Medical Education. To capitalize on this new sense of independence, the association established its *own* Council on Medical Education for the purpose of reviewing the credentials of eclectic colleges and accrediting them on the basis of a separate rating system. The committee consisted of N. A. Graves of Chicago, H. H. Helbing of St. Louis, T. D. Adlerman of Brooklyn, Paul Deogny of Milford, Nebraska, and Judge John Weld Peck of Cincinnati.[37]

From every region, particularly from the South and West, friends of eclectic medicine appealed to the trustees to resume classes, arguing that "the longer we wait, the harder it would become [to reopen]." Despite the lack of financial support from alumni, and the inability of the college to attract monies from foundations and individuals outside eclecticism, the pressure mounted for reopening the college.[38]

Not surprisingly, on July 2, 1931, having considered the appeals of alumni and the recommendations of the national association, the trustees responded with characteristic zeal. Only one member of the board dissented, questioning the advisibility of opening the college when there was no assurance that additional funds would be forthcoming. Undeterred, the trustees offered Byron H. Nellans the position of executive secretary at a salary of ten thousand dollars, contingent upon his ability to present a workable plan for opening the college in the fall.[39] Within a month, renovation of the building at 630 West Sixth Street had begun and, on the basis of Nellans's positive assurances, the board authorized him to matriculate a new freshman class. In supporting the decision, John Uri pledged ten thousand dollars a year for five years. Reminiscent of Phoenix rising from the ashes, the college admitted a freshman class in September 1931. Under its reorganization plan, the college provided instruction leading to the Doctor of Medicine and gave neither premedical nor postgraduate instruction.[40]

C. H. Carpenter, M.D., president of the Eclectic Medical Society of the State of California, gave an address praising the reopening of the college and expressing his loyalty and fraternalism. He urged eclectics to support not only their state and national societies but called attention to the fact that their alma mater needed financial support. Unfortunately, he observed, the graduates of the college were "greatly scattered" and few seemed to have any interest in advancing the eclectic cause.[41]

NELLANS'S INITIATION

Byron H. Nellans (1892–1949), the college's last dean and secretary, faced the burden of keeping the college alive on little more than promises and prayers. Born in Bloomingsburg, Indiana, in 1892, he graduated from the public schools, and matriculated at EMC in 1910. After graduating in 1914, he served residencies at Seton and St. Mary's hospitals before opening a practice in Cincinnati. For many years, he served as personal physician to John Uri Lloyd. From 1918 to 1934, he was professor of physical diagnosis and medicine; published articles in the *National Eclectic Medical Association Quarterly*; served as president, secretary, and treasurer of the Cincinnati Eclectic Medical Society and as president of the Ohio State Eclectic Medical Association; and in 1929 was elected president of the National Eclectic Medical Association. In March 1931, he became acting dean and later, after Eben B. Shewman (1876–1959) resigned following a brief term as dean in 1934–35, returned again as dean of the college, a position he held until 1939. Under his leadership, the school continued to seek endowment support, redesigned its curriculum, prepared an extensive self-study in anticipation of accreditation, and struggled with an

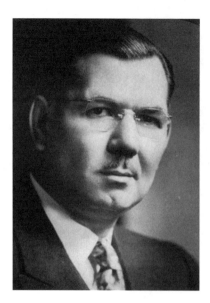

Byron H. Nellans, M.D. (1892–1949),
dean of EMC (1931–33, 1935–39).
Courtesy of the Lloyd Library
and Museum.

ever-dwindling budgetary base. Finally, as dean and secretary to the
college, he recommended the school's final closing and presided over
the dissolution of its real estate, equipment, and library. After closing
the college, he briefly became president of Lloyd Brothers Pharmacists, Inc., and, later, directed the Hamilton County Home and
Chronic Disease Hospital in Hartwell, Cincinnati.

In a candid analysis of eclectic medicine prepared by Nellans
shortly before becoming dean, he recounted the early history of eclecticism, focusing principally on the period from 1880, which marked
advances in surgery, bacteriology, and pathology by laboratory investigation. During this era, he observed, state legislatures and private
foundations had provided significant financial support to allopathic
schools; because of their "spectacular accomplishments," these schools
claimed title to most of the newer innovations in surgery and bacteriology. But in the last several years, Nellans noted that physicians of all
schools depended more on therapeutic methods than surgery and were
learning more about the effects of internal secretions, blood chemistry,
metabolism, and action of toxins and foreign proteins on functional or
physiological pathology. This, he felt, is where the eclectics should
have been focusing their attention. Here, too, was the natural domain
of the general practitioner. Unfortunately, eclectics had forfeited their

Eben Benjamin Shewman, M.D.
(1876–1959), dean of EMC (1934–35).
Courtesy of the Lloyd Library and
Museum.

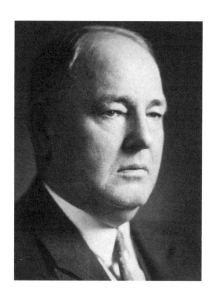

"golden opportunity for doing this research work for the last twenty years" and were thus in no position to benefit from recent discoveries. If they had written a new materia medica in the context of pathology and biochemistry and carried on their investigations in a more scientific manner, they would have become "leaders of medicine as well as practitioners of medicine, and we would have many great colleges because students would be eager to enter them." Since the eclectics had not taken the trouble to provide the means for investigation and research, they were left in the wake of allopathic medicine's more aggressive efforts. "Our Colleges have rapidly decreased, our journals are decreasing, our number of societies are decreasing, our numbers are decreasing because of lack of new graduates and deaths and retirements from the ranks," he concluded. The future was bleak. "Are we going to lie down and die?" He left his question unanswered.[42]

As dean and secretary, Nellans did the bidding of the college and the trustees but privately doubted the decision to reopen. Notwithstanding his reservations, Nellans's efforts to implement the school's reorganization plan resulted in licensing reciprocity, albeit provisional, in twenty-seven states. But the school remained handicapped by its lack of funding, and, equally important, it lacked approval by the AMA's Council on Medical Education. Without this,

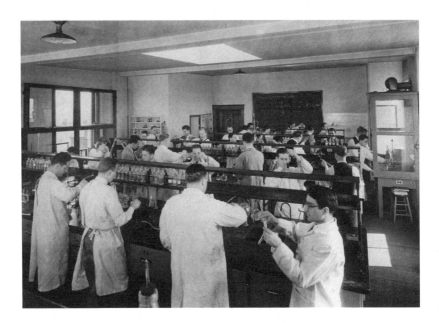

Students in pharmacy class, 1933. Courtesy of the Lloyd Library and Museum.

graduates could not be accepted by the tougher state licensing boards or, for that matter, obtain internships in approved hospitals.

Despite the school's decision to reopen in 1931, the American Medical Association maintained its classification status as "extinct" and refused to change its classification until the first student cohort completed its four-year course of study. Until then, Nellans could only convey to concerned parents and prospective students the college's intent to conduct itself "on the highest educational plane." In the meantime, he hoped that eclectic physicians would continue to send their sons and daughters to the college, and he encouraged applications from Jewish students forced to sidestep restrictive quotas in Eastern medical schools. Nellans's efforts were successful, as he proudly reported in August 1931 that the admissions committee was "swamped with applications."[43]

When the executive committee next met in March 1932, the freshman class was completing its first year of studies. With its advance to sophomore status came the challenge to meet increased expenditures

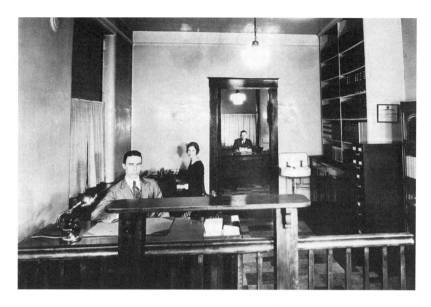

Second-floor administrative offices, 1933. The offices contained all student files, including grades and attendance records; minutes of regular and special meetings of the board of trustees and faculty; and textbooks and supplies. Courtesy of the Lloyd Library and Museum.

in biochemistry and physiology, which were "very much below the standard of modern teaching." Equally challenging was the required conversion of the existing operating and ampitheater rooms into pre-clinical laboratories in pathology, bacteriology, pharmacology, neuro-anatomy, and preventive medicine—not inconsequential costs.[44]

Nellans surprised the board a few months later by seeking permission to notify the Ohio State Medical Board that the college was ready for an inspection even though it had only just completed its first year. More surprising, he requested the board's permission to apply for membership in the Association of American Medical Colleges and ask for a review of the freshman class by its Committee on Inspection of Medical Colleges. When asked what the college hoped to gain by the inspection, Treasurer Beaman replied that, while not optimistic the AAMC would act favorably on the application, he intended to test the association's willingness to review the college. But Nellans also hinted at other, more serious motives behind the request. It seems that many of the faculty, certainly the few who had been educated in regular schools, but even some who had graduated from the college, were reluctant to teach for any length of time unless the college could obtain a more favorable rating. Equally disturbing, Dean Arthur C. Bachmeyer of the University of Cincinnati refused to permit his faculty to serve as adjunct professors to the college or as hospital residents unless the college received a favorable rating. Given the seriousness of these reservations, the board had no recourse but to support the request.[45]

The lack of a rating by the Council on Medical Education carried serious implications, including the inability of students to obtain loans for their education. A letter to the college administration from the board of education of the Methodist Episcopal Church indicated that EMC students were ineligible to obtain loans because the college had less than a class-A ranking. "An inviolable requirement for borrowing while in attendance at a Medical School," wrote the loan clerk to a prospective applicant of EMC, "is that the institution be rated as class 'A' by the accrediting Council. Unfortunately for your present plans, it would seem that the Eclectic Medical College does not meet this condition and candidates therein enrolled would be ineligible for aid from the fund."[46]

To assist in its approval efforts, the college established a legal advisory committee chaired by Judge John Weld Peck, a close friend of John Uri Lloyd. Known for his political acumen and his wide range of influential friends, Peck instructed Nellans and Shewman on how best to approach the Ohio State Medical Board and how to respond to queries from the Association of American Medical Colleges and the Council on Medical Education. In particular, Peck tutored the two administrators on how to negotiate with Dr. Harold Rypins, M.D., secretary to the New York State Board of Medical Examiners, the sole inspector of medical colleges for the state, who reputedly was within the "innermost circle" of the AAMC and AMA.[47]

The financial problems of the college worsened with the depression. Had John Uri not agreed in 1933 to advance a portion of his gift money earlier than intended, and had Judge Thomas Vaughn Morrow (a newly elected member of the board and a descendant of the school's first dean) not agreed to intervene on behalf of the college for a loan, the college might have closed earlier. Even so, the college was twelve thousand dollars overdrawn, and Beaman and Nellans were able to draw only a portion of their own salaries. Sadly, the Eclectic Education Loyalty Fund had received a mere $1,695 in pledges, of which only $542.50 had been paid. The college's total operating expenses amounted to less than what the University of Cincinnati Medical School expended in a single department.[48]

CLASS OF 1935

The members of the class of 1935 who entered EMC in September 1931, came from ten different states and were immediately immersed in H. W. MacMillan's grinding course of anatomy, F. J. Andress's biochemistry, F. A. Fischer's histology, and Cloyce Wilson's eclectic materia medica.[49] Gone were the days of boisterous class rivalries, hazing, and pranks, as students embarked on the business of their education with total seriousness.[50] Of thirty-five original students, only twenty-eight entered the second year. Reasons for the attrition included poor grades and transfers to other medical schools. By the third year the class, which had now dwindled to twenty-two, separated into two groups to facilitate clinical clerkships. Union Bethel Clinic and its outpatient department provided the clinical experience for junior-year instruction.[51] In existence for ninety-three years, the clinic served an average of a thousand patients annually. Contact with patients as well as the laboratory and apparatus that permitted a complete workup of patients brought added impetus to the students' enthusiasm. In addition to clinical work, the class received lectures from the clinicians and professors.[52]

With the advent of the fourth year, the class of 1935 lost another two students. Nevertheless, spirits ran high, due principally to the decision of Cincinnati General Hospital to mix EMC students in with those from the University of Cincinnati. Internships and state board examinations were uppermost on the minds of students, and, gradually, as the year progressed, members of the class found positions in various hospitals.[53]

Of the first class of twenty that graduated under the reorganization plan on June 7, 1935, eighteen passed the Ohio State Board Examination and were placed in approved hospitals. At the time, the college boasted a total of 132 students (thirty-one seniors, twenty-three juniors, thirty-four sophomores, and forty-four freshmen) receiving instruction and training from more than one hundred members of the faculty, most of whom served without pay.[54]

In his notification for the 1935–36 session, Treasurer Beaman informed students that, besides an annual tuition fee of three hundred dollars payable in full or half for the fall semester, there was a fee of five dollars for late registrants (plus fifty cents for each day of delinquency), and students failing to pay after the fourth week faced disenrollment. He expected each student to come with a fully equipped microscope and all necessary medical texts. The college also instituted a breakage fee of five dollars; a laboratory fee of fifteen dollars for physiology, pathology, biochemistry, bacteriology, and pharmacology; a clinic fee of fifteen dollars; a library fee of one dollar; a fee of five dollars for every supplemental examination taken for the removal of a "condition"; and a graduation fee of ten dollars.[55] As if the higher cost of education was not enough, the college terminated one of its faculty members who, it was learned, had been guilty of pawning student microscopes for cash.[56]

The faculty were well aware that the college represented a last chance for many students seeking medical training. In a meeting of the executive committee in 1935, Nellans noted the applications from students requesting to repeat a freshman year or who were asking admission to advanced standing after having dropped out of another medical college because of poor grades. Fearing that a continuation of this practice would jeopardize the school's standing with the Council on Medical Education, the committee approved a new policy prohibiting admission or advanced standing to any student identified as special or irregular.[57]

Under the new rules, the admissions committee endeavored to walk a narrow line when it came to marginal students, a situation that proved troubling, since it sometimes affected the sons and daughters of former graduates. One 1905 graduate who practiced in Durant, Oklahoma, intended to enroll both his daughter and son-in-law in the 1934–35 session. Knowing that his son-in-law lacked sufficient hours in chemistry and physics, he asked Marquis E. Daniel, chairman of the reciprocity committee of the Texas State Board of Medical Examiners, to write Dean Nellans on behalf of the applicants, promising that the young couple would dedicate their lives to eclecticism in the Southwest and intimating that the father intended "to do something in the not distant future for the college at least to the extent of paying for some life insurance for the benefit of the college."[58] Nellans reluctantly informed the father that, while his daughter met admission standards for the freshman class, his son-in-law failed to meet the school's basic science requirements. "This College is working, at the present time, under a re-organization plan," he wrote. "Every move that we make is being carefully watched. We would be subject to severe criticism and we would not be complying with our pre-medical requirements if we were to waive so many hours credit on this young man." Nellans apologized to the father and offered to reserve a place for his son-in-law in the class of 1935, provided he completed the needed hours at a college or university.[59]

On hearing the news, the father wrote Daniel and complained bitterly of Nellans's response. Daniel, who had a clearer understanding of the changing medical scene, made every effort to explain the dean's decision.

> My dear boy, Dr. Nellans' decision is not his as an individual. It is present day Eclecticism's decision. He [Nellans] is only Eclecticism's hired hand. As I told you plainly the college must live up to a fixed standard to be able *to live at all*—a standard the educational world must recognize as reputable and yet this standard is NO HIGHER than that of any other reputable college. I tell you again that every reputable college in this country EXACTS a standard just as high which standard is that of the American Medical College Association [sic], or else they are falsifying the published requirement they are supposed to live up to.[60]

A year later, after the son-in-law removed his deficiencies in the basic sciences, the couple matriculated in the 1935 class. The son-in-law graduated in 1939 while his wife withdrew following her junior year for health reasons.[61]

The initial years of the college's reopening represented a time of cautious optimism punctuated by financial embarrassment, ever-increasing demands by the American Medical Association, and a gradual feeling of hopelessness for the cause of eclecticism. As Nellans would soon discover, the pressures finally to close the school would come not just from forces outside eclecticism, but from the ranks of EMC's own faculty and students.

– CHAPTER SIX –

Denouement

O N THE ADVICE OF Judge John Weld Peck of the college's Legal Advisory Committee, Dean Byron Nellans appeared before the Ohio State Medical Board on January 9, 1934, and successfully argued EMC's case for provisional approval. Several months later, eclectics N. A. Graves, M.D., of Chicago and T. D. Adlerman, M.D., of Brooklyn, representing the Council on Medical Education of the National Eclectic Medical Association, made a site visit. Based on their advice and recommendation, the association at its meeting in Detroit voted to give the college a class-A rating. However meritorious this rating was felt among eclectics, the association's classification made little impression on the Ohio licensing board and hospitals and no impression at all on the American Medical Association or the Association of American Medical Colleges.[1]

In June 1934 came news that a New York hospital refused to permit an EMC graduate to intern because of the school's "extinct" classification. Nellans immediately appealed to the director of the hospital explaining that, according to AMA policies, the college could not register for reclassification until June 1935, following graduation of its first senior class; the director listened but refused to reinstate the intern.[2] The school's precarious condition became quickly evident as students from New York and New Jersey, intent on practicing in their home states, learned of the hospital's action. "Whether or not we will be able to practice in our own State," wrote one concerned graduate in a letter to Nellans, "is an important item in our lives." He and other classmates repeatedly asked the dean for information on the subject. None was forthcoming.[3]

In a letter to Nellans, one New York student reported a conversation with Harold Rypins, M.D., secretary to the New York State Board

of Medical Examiners and member of the National Board of Medical
Examiners, who had informed him that EMC was no longer registered
in New York and that this decision had been reported to the school
administration. When the student defended the quality of the school,
Rypins interjected that the student was only in his preclinical years
and could not speak for any hospital experience. Rypins went on to say
that access to Cincinnati's general hospital had been wholly inadequate. "The way he expressed it," wrote the student, was that "we are
'parasites' of the hospital." The student explained how he had tried to
correct Rypins. "Doctor," he said, "I am sure everything will turn out
all right because our school is as good as any in the country." Rypins
reportedly responded with a big smile and the remark: "Good luck to
you boy." Fearing that he had missed something in the communication, the student asked Nellans what Rypins meant by his reference to
a report.[4] Obviously, Nellans had not communicated to students the
contents of the report or the change in status of the college.

In a last disappointing effort to improve its endowment, the college hired Dr. John J. Sutter of Lima, Ohio, as fundraiser. Together
with Nellans and Shewman, Sutter visited Jewish alumni in New York
and New Jersey seeking endowment funds. The trip turned out to be a
crushing defeat for the college; while the New York and New Jersey
alumni desired to see the school continue, they were unwilling to provide financial support or even be associated with it. Having used EMC
to obtain entrance into medicine, they now preferred to conceal their
eclectic origins and practice as regulars.[5]

The Survey

Recognizing that the school could no longer draw students from New
York without recognition by the state's board of regents, the trustees
directed Shewman and Nellans to prepare a response to a nationwide
survey developed by the AMA's Council on Medical Education, a
survey begun in 1933 and made with the cooperation of the Association of American Medical Colleges and the Federation of State Medical Boards of the United States. In it, the college provided a wealth
of information, including the composition of its board of trustees,
committee and governance structure, policies and procedures, faculty,
clinical sites, curriculum, library, staff support, and finances.

At the time of the survey, the trustees included Charles S. Amidon, M.D., surgeon; Charles W. Beaman, M.D., pediatrician; William P. Best, M.D., general practitioner; Charles R. Campbell, M.D., county commissioner; J. Stewart Hagen, M.D., surgeon; Rev. Jesse Halsey, pastor, Seventh Presbyterian Church; John Uri Lloyd, pharmacist, scientist, philanthropist, and author; Judge Thomas V. Morrow, common pleas court; William Nelson Mundy, M.D., general practitioner; Byron H. Nellans, M.D., secretary to the college; Frank H. Shaffer, L.L.B., member of Peck, Shaffer and Williams; Eben B. Shewman, M.D., surgeon; and Rev. Louis G. Hoek, pastor, Swedenborgian Church.[6] Besides their annual and special meetings, the trustees served on Executive, Finance and Real Estate, and Hospital Committees as well as on several ad hoc committees, the most important being the Legal Advisory Committee chaired by Judge John Weld Peck. Eben Shewman, professor of surgery and dean for a brief period, divided his time between the college and private practice, while his chief executive officer, Byron H. Nellans, devoted his time exclusively to the management of the college. As dean, Shewman wrote reports to the board of trustees, presided over faculty meetings, met with the faculty council, and served as chairman of the hospital committee, conferring regularly with the superintendent of the Cincinnati General Hospital and the director of the Hamilton County Tuberculosis Sanatorium regarding the instruction and curriculum for junior and senior students.[7]

The faculty consisted of three professors emeritus; thirty professors; fifteen associate professors; twenty assistant professors; thirty instructors; twenty assistants; and ten special lecturers. Their committees included Administration, Admissions, Microscopes, Preceptors, Internships, and Promotions. All appointments to these committees were made by the trustees upon the recommendation of a Faculty Council consisting of department heads and presided over by the dean. The council addressed longterm planning, purchases, curricular matters, and day-to-day administrative issues. Support staff included five secretaries, two part-time and two full-time record clerks, a registrar and director of admissions, and several clinic directors.[8]

Faculty were hired on year-to-year contracts, with reappointment contingent upon quality and ability. Selection followed personal interviews, a review of the applicant's statement as to character and morals, college and graduate training, teaching experience, professional memberships, and research. There was no formal policy on tenure and, since faculty relied principally on their private practice for income, the college made no provision for retirement or other benefits.[9]

Of the thirty-five faculty members who completed the survey, twenty-five were graduates of the college. Of the ten who came with other credentials, seven were graduates of the University of Cincinnati, one was from Ohio State, one from the University of Michigan, and one from the Cincinnati College of Dental Surgery. Of the total faculty, four were full-time salaried instructors and two were administrators. The remainder divided their time between teaching and private practice. Only three of the thirty-five had worked in the clinics of Berlin, Vienna, or Budapest.[10] Eight were members of the American Medical Association and known as the "allopathic minority" within the college.[11]

At the time of the survey, the college consisted of the building at 628–30 West Sixth Street, which had a replacement value of $125,000. It housed the administrative offices of the school as well as the laboratories for anatomy, biochemistry, physiology, pathology, bacteriology, preventive medicine, pharmacology, and materia medica. In addition, the building contained a museum, medical art department, library, recitation and lecture rooms, and an assembly hall.[12] The library had an annual budget of two thousand dollars, and a collection of 3,627 books and eighty periodicals. It was supported by a librarian and an assistant and was open every day of the week from nine until five. In addition, students had access to the Lloyd Library with its collection of 60,000 books and 30,000 pamphlets, the Cincinnati General Hospital Library with its 42,771 books and 31,822 pamphlets, and the Cincinnati Public Library with its 6,500 volumes.[13]

The survey explained that juniors had access to the Hamilton County Tuberculosis Sanitorium, between Price Hill and Westwood, six miles from the college, along with the outpatient department and dispensary of the Union Bethel Clinic. The sanitorium operated under a lease from the city and all its 639 beds were available for teaching purposes. However, the sanitorium staff, like the staff of the Cincinnati Hospital, was appointed by the board of directors of the University of Cincinnati, which meant that EMC faculty could hold no staff privileges.[14] Seniors had access to Longview Hospital for the treatment of nervous and mental students and Cincinnati General Hospital. The latter, located at Burnet Avenue, three miles from the college,

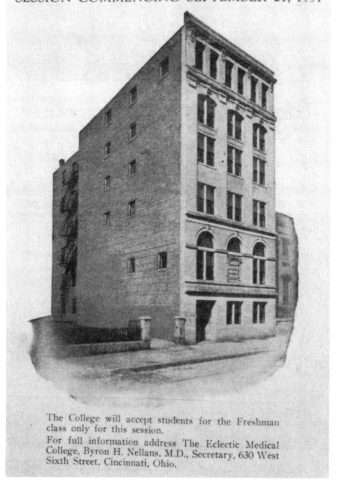

The Eclectic Medical College
Cincinati, Ohio
ANNOUNCE THE EIGHTY-SEVENTH ANNUAL SESSION COMMENCING SEPTEMBER 21, 1931

The College will accept students for the Freshman class only for this session.

For full information address The Eclectic Medical College, Byron H. Nellans, M.D., Secretary, 630 West Sixth Street, Cincinnati, Ohio.

Eclectic Medical College, 630 West Sixth Street, Cincinnati, 1931. Courtesy of the Lloyd Library and Museum.

had 860 beds available (16,777 admissions in 1934). Senior-year medical instruction was open to EMC students; but, since no EMC faculty member had staff privileges at the hospital, all supervision was done by the faculty and staff of the University of Cincinnati Medical School. Alternatively, junior and senior classes had limited access to Bethesda, St. Mary's, and Deaconess Hospitals, whose staff physicians included numerous eclectics. By the standards of the day, these latter three hospitals were marginal at best, with small and often obsolete facilities and equipment.[15]

Following completion of the survey, Harold Rypins, M.D., visited the college on March 6–9, 1935. Since the first class had graduated under the reorganization plan, Rypins was invited to validate its qualifictions for licensing. In his written report received on May 7, he informed the college that the New York State Board of Medical Examiners would continue to refuse recognition to the school and thus deny reciprocity. According to Rypins, a thorough inspection of the college revealed that it "does not have adequate equipment and resources, that it does not have suitable hospital and clinical facilities, that it does not maintain an adequate medical library and that it does not have a sufficient number of full-time salaried instructors giving their entire time to professional instruction, and thus does not meet four of the seven requirements of the Board of Regents, for the recognition of a medical school." While Nellans thought the college could successfully challenge Rypins's claim of inadequacy in the areas of equipment and library materials, he admitted that the college could not argue that suitable hospital and clinical facilities existed or, for that matter, that a sufficient number of salaried instructors gave their entire time to professional instruction.[16]

Rypins's report was followed in June 1935 by a letter from William D. Cutter, secretary to the AMA's Council on Medical Education, which contained an abstract of his findings during a site visit completed at the same time as the Rypins visit. Cutter informed the board that the council voted not to approve the college because of improper organization of its board of trustees (too many department heads served on the board), the lack of adequate hospital and clinical facilities, an insufficient number of full-time salaried instructors, and the lack of faculty research and space for carrying it out.[17]

Of the deficiencies identified in the findings, Nellans believed the college was most vulnerable in its lack of adequate hospital facilities.

According to the report, which Nellans read to the board, the fourth-year students were assigned to the Cincinnati General Hospital for only a half-day. Since "no member of the faculty of the Eclectic school holds a position on the staff of the Hospital, the school has no control of the activities of its students,—thus 'farming out' its students to another organization . . . flagrantly evades its own responsibilities and obligations."[18]

In responding to the advice of Cutter and Dean H. G. Weiskotten of Syracuse University College of Medicine (the two authors of the written findings), the trustees agreed to change their composition and revise the college's curriculum to the extent that finances permitted. Shewman, Beaman, and Nellans, the respective heads of the departments of surgery, pediatrics, and medicine, resigned from the board. Shewman also resigned as dean of the faculty and was replaced by Nellans, a favorite of the students and alumni. Consistent with the recommendations of the external reviewers, Nellans became a full-time salaried dean. In addition, the college hired two new full-time salaried instructors and one full-time technician. However, no money was available for additional salaried instructors in the departments of physiology and anatomy.[19]

News of the findings of Cutter, Weiskotten, and Rypins devastated the morale of faculty and students alike, and they were further dismayed by a report that the New York regents had refused to permit a recent EMC graduate to take the state medical examination. Requested by the student's attorney to join suit to combat the decision, the college trustees saw no recourse but to remain silent; the student subsequently lost his case.[20] Nellans's efforts to obtain staff privileges at Cincinnati General Hospital stalled, and requests to discuss relationships with the Cincinnati General Hospital and with Alfred Friedlander, M.D., the new dean of the University of Cincinnati Medical School, were met with stony silence.[21]

Most disheartening to students was the news that EMC graduates were no longer eligible for internships in approved hospitals. The catalyst for this decision was the Council on Medical Education's warning to hospitals that approval depended on their refusal to accept graduates of class-B medical schools. Following the council's edict, worried hospital administrators began asking eclectic interns to resign their posts.[22] Nellans, having accepted a new freshman class of forty-three students for the 1935–36 session, and giving instruction to thirty-one seniors, twenty-three juniors, and thirty-five sophomores, doubted that any of these students could receive class-A hospital and clinical experiences.

On October 5, 1935, not long after the site visits, the Council on Medical Education reported that, nationally, medical schools had revealed certain common weaknesses. These included increased enrollment without a corresponding increase in personnel and instructional facilities, insufficient correlation between clinical and laboratory knowledge, and sectarianism's negative effect on medical education and advances in the medical sciences. The council resolved that the number of students in each medical school should "not exceed the number that can be adequately taught with the laboratory, library and clinical facilities available and for whom a sufficiently large and competent teaching staff is provided"; that after July 1, 1938, the council would no longer publish a list of approved two-year medical schools; and, finally, that after July 1, 1938, the council would no longer carry sectarian schools of medicine on its approved list.[23]

In response to the council's notification, the board of the New York Homeopathic College and Flowers Hospital changed the institution's name to the New York Medical College and the Fifth Avenue Hospital, thereby relinquishing its long-held sectarian status. In reporting this information to the executive committee in December 1935, Nellans stated that the decision by the homeopaths to "give up their birthright" seriously affected the future of EMC. He then advised the committee to "proceed with extreme caution" in deciding to matriculate a new freshmen class in the fall. Unless EMC could be "very materially strengthened," it was better to close enrollments and seek affiliation with another university.[24]

On January 14, 1936, the board of trustees called a special meeting to address issues vital to the future of the college and "to the very existence of [eclecticism in] American medicine." In his report to the board, Nellans reminded the trustees that H. M. Platter, M.D., secretary of the State Medical Board of Ohio, had notified the college on January 26, 1935, of the board's unanimous decision to grant provisional recognition to the college but had urged certain improvements be made effective "at the earliest possible moment." Specifically, the secretary encouraged the trustees to move forward with their plans for new construction and for ensuring better supervision of students in the Cincinnati General Hospital. Neither seemed possible. Since all medical colleges in the country were undergoing a general inspection by the Council on Medical Education, the secretary indicated that the board would look at the progress of the college in 1938, specifically at the problem areas noted by Cutter and Weiskotten. Nellans made it clear that the Ohio board would base its final decision on the college's compliance with the recommendations of the Council on Medical Education.[25]

Nellans then reviewed the council's decision to remove sectarian medical colleges from its approved list of schools. This decision, irrespective of facilities or resources, meant that the college had no chance of being registered in New York and most other states. This also meant that internships in approved hospitals for the present senior class, let alone future students, would be impossible. Nellans reported "a marked feeling of unrest" among the students, who were beginning to realize the full import of these decisions upon their future livelihood.

> I am very much discouraged and am of the opinion that the day of sectarian medicine in America has come to the end. The fact that the College, with its present finances and resources can not meet the present requirements of the Council on Medical Education, the fact that they will no longer carry schools of sectarian medicine on their approved list, the fact that we cannot obtain satisfactory interneships [sic] for our graduates, and, last but not least the very fact that we can not meet the educational program and attain the high educational standards that we ourselves have set up, leads me to believe that we should give immediate concern to honorably discharging the moral obligations we owe to the present student body. We certainly should not matriculate a Freshman class this fall unless a definite solution is found for our present problems, and the future of the College unreservedly assured. . . . I am of the opinion that the Eclectic Medical College of Cincinnati, as presently constituted, can no longer continue as an undergraduate school. Please believe me, when I state that this school is really a part of my life and I am grieved and deeply moved to see this worthy section of American Medicine placed in such an unfavorable position. Our traditions are honorable, our aims are honorable, yet today, there is a definite, powerful organization opposing sectarian medicine in this country.[26]

Nellans concluded his report by recommending three options for consideration: first, an affiliation with Xavier University or the YMCA that would include a chair of eclectic materia medica and medicine and thus perpetuate the purpose of the school; second, surrendering the charter to some other "worthy institution" and use any resources for the endowment of a chair of eclectic materia medica and medicine; or third, notifying the Council on Medical Education that the college would accept no more classes and ask its support in enabling the college to graduate the presently enrolled students by admitting them to approved hospitals for internship and thereby "honorably discharge our moral obligations" to the student body.[27]

On January 31, in yet another special meeting, the trustees considered a set of five recommendations brought forward by Nellans. Each motion carried.

1. *Resolved:* "That the Board of Trustees of the Eclectic Medical College do not accept a freshman class for matriculation for the 1936–37 Session and that the Dean be instructed to so notify those applying for admission."

2. *Resolved:* "That the Board of Trustees of the Eclectic Medical College terminate undergraduate instruction at the graduation of the present freshman class of 1939, i.e., to complete the undergraduate medical education of all students enrolled at the present time who maintain a satisfactory scholastic standing; thus honorably discharging our moral obligation to them; and further, that no students be accepted for matriculation to advanced standing."

3. *Resolved:* "That the Dean be instructed to reorganize the faculty and personnel of the various departments of the College to conform with the above program and that final action must be authorized by the Executive Committee of the Board of Trustees, acting upon the advice of the Finance Committee."

4. *Resolved:* "That the Secretary report the decision of the Board of Trustees of the Eclectic Medical College to the faculty, student body and alumni of the College, the Councils on Medical Education of the National Eclectic Medical Association and the American Medical Association, state medical boards where the College is recognized at the present time, and such other organizations and individuals as may be deemed necessary and proper."

5. *Resolved:* "That a committee of three be appointed by the Board of Trustees to study the ways and means of establishing under the Board's direction a scientific research foundation. The purpose and aims of this foundation would be to advance the science and art of medicine and improve the public health. It would also direct the study and development of the Eclectic practice of Medicine and the Eclectic Materia Medica by scientific investigation with emphasis on its pharmacology, physiological action and clinical application. Thus the principals of the Eclectic practice of Medicine would be continued."[28]

On March 20, 1936, Secretary Campbell informed the State Medical Board of Ohio that the trustees had resolved not to accept a freshman class for matriculation for the 1936–37 session and that the college would end all medical instruction with the graduation of the present freshman class in 1939.[29]

Immediately following this action, Nellans terminated several members of the teaching staff and embarked on a retrenchment program that utilized faculty members on a need basis but closed their contracts once classes ended. He also began selling equipment and apparatus no longer required in the program. In addition, he traveled to Chicago to meet with Cutter and inquire about the AMA's position toward the college's status now that it had closed admissions. Cutter informed him that the Council on Medical Education refused to modify its ruling, which meant that the final three classes would be denied internships in approved hospitals. The New York regents refused to reconsider their action as well.[30]

Nellans received harsh criticism from older eclectics for his recommendation to close the college. Their remarks hurt him deeply, and in numerous letters to friends he attempted to justify the recommendation and its implications. He revealed in a moment of candor that the trustees had been "foolish" to reopen the college in 1931 with the limited funds on hand. He also believed the school could not operate on the fringes of medical respectability, unrecognized by the AMA's Council on Medical Education. Either the college existed on its own weight and reputation or it needed to close. What hurt him most was the lack of loyalty among the college's New York and New Jersey alumni. "It appears that once they receive their diploma they lose all interest in the school," Nellans wrote despondently.[31]

In explaining his actions to longtime friend Herbert T. Cox, the dean observed that medical education had undergone enormous changes and that the college was simply not in a position to compete with those that were more richly endowed or held municipal, state, or university affiliations. "We think it much better to honorably close," he wrote, "than to attempt to run a 'wild-cat' institution." With, in his estimation, only 2 percent of the alumni loyal to the college, and with only forty-one physicians registered for the annual eclectic meeting in Ohio, eclecticism as a school of thought was perilously close to extinction. As evidence of this, Nellans pointed out that alumni were refusing to send their sons and daughters to the institution, knowing it was a handicap for them to attend a school that was not council-approved. "I realize that this is a pretty black picture to paint," Nellans concluded, but "many of those who have been loyal for so many years are weary of the fight." Since the income from tuition no longer paid the cost of a medical doctor's education, and since the college lacked the ability to make up the deficit, there was no other option but to close.[32]

Friends of Nellans tried to boost his spirits by praising the heroic efforts he had taken to reestablish the college and by complimenting him for his tireless work. In assessing why so few eclectics seemed willing to help the college, William P. Best, M.D., president of the National Eclectic Medical Association, concluded that the majority of eclectics were of a "humble type" and in no manner prepared to meet its financial needs.[33] Theodore Alderman, editor and manager of the *National Eclectic Medical Association Quarterly*, urged Nellans to ignore the criticisms since the college had died an honorable death, unlike others that were attempting mergers with naturopaths, chiropractors, and other "paths." For Adlerman, those efforts represented an attempt to enter the medical field "through the watercloset doors."[34] Nellans's colleague, A. Harry Crum, M.D., remarked that his inability to perpetuate the Eclectic Medical College could in no way be interpreted as a personal failure. American medicine had made great strides in the past fifty years, and the fault lay with Nellans's predecessors who had failed to keep abreast. Nellans's own efforts to restore the college to a high plane, which necessitated his relinquishing a lucrative personal practice, testified to his devotion to the "cause of Eclecticism."[35] Nevertheless, eclectics west of the Mississippi and from the South wanted him to carry on regardless of the consequences and provided him with any number of suggestions for saving the college. Nellans reported than "none of them [suggestions] appear to have any merit."[36]

AFFILIATIONS

The last three years of the college were difficult ones for the dean and trustees. Money remained tight and several members of the board secured private bank loans in order for the school to meet its payroll. Nellans himself had to settle for less than his stipulated salary and efforts to sell equipment fell woefully short of expectations.[37] By the end of 1937, barely $3,400 had been recovered from the sale of equipment. Beaman and Nellans blamed the small sum on depreciation and the difficult financial state of the country. Eventually, the trustees authorized Nellans to give the unsold equipment to those doctors who for years had donated their services to the college.[38] Nellans continued to confer with administrators at Xavier University and the University of Cincinnati on the possibility that one of them might take over the college. These talks, including the possibility of establishing a chair of eclectic materia medica, dragged on for months without resolution.[39]

In December 1935, Shewman informed the executive committee that the YMCA, which for years had rented rooms for students in its facilities a few blocks from the college, had expressed an interest in acquiring the school. With the future of the college in doubt and with no other affiliation worked out, Louis G. Hoeck, president of the trustees and chair of the executive committee, appointed a subcommittee to explore the proposition. The subcommittee subsequently met with Judge Robert N. Gorman of the first judicial district of Ohio, representing the executive committee of YMCA's educational department (which administered a Law School, Commerce School, Business School, and a Night High School in Cincinnati) to explain the full implications—fiscal and academic—for obtaining an "A" classification. Despite the grim picture portrayed by the subcommittee, Judge Gorman proposed that the YMCA take over and operate EMC, thus ensuring that the eclectic method of teaching would continue.[40] In urging approval of the proposal, he explained that the YMCA was in a much better political position nationally to address the policy issues and demands of the American Medical Association. He recognized that the other YMCA-sponsored schools were not sectarian, meaning that men and women of "all creeds" were eligible to join their classes, but that the policy would be waived in this instance and the college would become known as the "YMCA Eclectic Medical College." Gorman further stipulated that the present trustees would continue to govern the college for at least three years and, thereafter, a majority of the trustees would be elected from the college's alumni. He also desired Nellans to continue as dean but stated that no plan could be successful if it resulted in a large deficit. His intent was to make the college self-sustaining within a few years of acquisition. Not long after making his offer, Gorman realized the full measure of financial risk as well as the implications of the AMA's decision to no longer carry sectarian schools on its approved list after 1938 and withdrew his offer.[41]

In November of 1938, there was discussion of transferring the library collection to George S. Sperti, director of the Institutum Divi Thomae, a basic science laboratory on Mt. Washington in Cincinnati. In return, Sperti promised to provide adequate space for research on the materia medica and support fellowships for young scholars interested in eclectic pharmacology.[42] Before negotiations progressed very far, the board received a letter from John Thomas Lloyd, the son of John Uri who had formed his own company, the John T. Lloyd Laboratories, Inc., to carry on the work of his father. In his letter, John T. proposed that the school's library, as well as the student records, be moved to his laboratories with the understanding that the books would be properly cataloged to support research on plant remedies stressing the eclectic materia medica. As for student records, they would be available to proper officers of the college and to licensing boards.[43] Aware of the legacy left by John Uri, the board found itself unable to refuse the offer, and at its May 20, 1938, meeting, voted to transfer the library and records to the John T. Lloyd Laboratories, Inc.[44]

In one last desperate gamble, Nellans met with a Dr. Kring of Ft. Wayne, Indiana, representing the National Executive Committee of the Odd Fellows of the United States, to consider whether the college might become part of a university that the Odd Fellows were considering founding. Nothing came of the meeting and no action resulted.[45]

UNFRIENDLY PERSUASION

Recognizing the cost of maintaining the college building at 630 West Sixth Street was no longer justified for the remaining students, Nellans leased the third-floor offices at 17 East Eighth Street in a building owned by two of the faculty. In January 1937, the college, with its files and remaining apparatus, moved into its smaller quarters.[46]

Junior-year instruction continued at the Union Bethel Clinic at 501–5 East Third Street, where students worked in three groups: medicine, surgery, and specialties. Each group worked eleven weeks in a section before rotating so that all students ended the year with the same clinical instruction. In accordance with a gentleman's agreement, the college staffed the clinic, furnished all supplies and equipment needs, and was responsible for the supervision of the students in the laboratory. The students' work in the various departments of the clinic was carefully supervised and graded and the remaining faculty faithfully gave the prescribed courses of lectures in the curriculum.[47]

For senior-year students, Nellans negotiated an arrangement with Dean Friedlander of the University of Cincinnati Medical School to provide instruction in medicine, pediatrics, and surgery. Aside from the fact that their attendance was not checked, EMC students enjoyed most of the same privileges as the university's medical students. In only one instance did a medical department refuse to assign individual cases to EMC students. And where the college was unable to obtain faculty to cover a specific area, Nellans himself took over the teaching.[48]

In the last two years of instruction, Nellans spent much of his energy locating schools so that his students could transfer. Writing David V. McCauley, S.J., dean of Georgetown University School of Medicine in March 1937, he reported that the Council on Medical Education had ruled that EMC students were now eligible (on account of the college's decision to close) for advanced standing in approved medical schools. Presumably Nellans had concluded that the AMA was prepared to credit the graduates of the college for their work. Actually, the association had decided to credit the graduates only after the official order of dissolution had been made by the trustees to Secretary of State John E. Sweeney of Ohio. This had not yet happened and, in fact, would not occur until March 17, 1942. In the meantime, the students, the dean, and the faculty labored hard to arrange for internships and transfers based on this incorrect assumption.[49]

In a letter to Nellans dated July 16, 1937, a student reported a conversation with Dr. William A. Pearson, dean of the Hahnemann Medical College and Hospital of Philadelphia. Although the dean was "favorably disposed" to accepting the student as a transfer, he feared repercussion from the AMA. In his conversation with the dean, the student gave assurances that Nellans had received a letter from the AMA's Council on Medical Education to the effect that students could transfer to a class-A school provided the receiving institution was willing to recognize the student's work. Since the student could not produce a copy of the letter, Pearson refused the request. "I feel that a photostatic copy of that letter would do much to benefit my cause," the student wrote in his letter to Nellans.[50] Such a letter is not in the files of the college or in Nellans's effects; nor is there a record of Nellans having written Pearson regarding the supposed letter. There is, however, a letter from Dean Pearson to Nellans informing him of his talk with the student and with a member of the Pennsylvania state legislature. Pearson said he had advised the student to complete his medical program at EMC since he would then be eligible to obtain his license to practice in Ohio. As for the student's hospital internship, the dean offered his help to secure an appointment in "one of the many good hospitals not approved by the American Medical Association." However, Hahnemann Medical College could provide neither. "It is exceedingly unfortunate that medical colleges and hospitals approved by the AMA cannot assist your students and graduates without running the risk of endangering their status," Pearson wrote.[51]

Nellans received numerous letters from worried students and graduates seeking clarification on the issue. One wrote the dean asking whether his grades were adequate enough for him to transfer to a "recognized medical school and in that way obtain approved recognition."[52] Nellans replied that, to date, none of the seniors had been accepted as transfers since medical schools were reluctant to take them for one year's instruction before granting the degree. "My advice to you," he wrote, "would be to return here next week for registration, take your last year with us and graduate next June, take your Ohio State Medical Board Examination and then your status in this state is the same as any other physician." He assured the student that the internship question "is gradually being cleared up" and promised to place him in a "good hospital" and perhaps even an approved one.[53] The student followed Nellans's advice and graduated a year later.[54]

Some letters in the school's file were from graduates imploring Nellans and the faculty for help; others were copies of originals sent to the graduates by particular hospitals. One such letter in 1937 from C. H.

Young, M.D., of Little Rock, Arkansas, explained to a recent graduate the political situation in the state and the difficulties that eclectics were having in obtaining hospital internships. "The chances are very slim," he wrote, considering that the University of Arkansas School of Medicine with its forty to sixty students had first choice of any hospital in Arkansas. Even the Missouri Pacific Hospital, which lacked a class-A status, had applications for internships from students at the Arkansas School of Medicine. Young indicated that he himself had interned in the hospital at a time when the chief surgeon was a close friend and supporter of eclecticism. But times had changed and the new chief surgeon was on the staff of the Arkansas School of Medicine and naturally preferred his own students for interns.[55]

Young, himself an official of the Arkansas Eclectic State Medical Board, encouraged the graduate to apply to the Missouri Pacific Hospital. He also urged him to apply to the Baptist State Hospital in Little Rock and to use Young as a reference. "Tell them that I visited your school on two occasions; know personally many of the faculty, including Dr. Nellans and ask them to give the students consideration. Here would be your only chance. The hospitals here and the School [University of Arkansas Medical School] gets into controversies every now and then and some student that agrees to intern . . . fails to show up, leaving them short; then it would be that you might get a chance."[56]

Arkansas at that time did not require doctors to have a hospital internship before taking the Arkansas Eclectic State Medical Board exam; they had only to pass the basic science exam and then the medical exam before entering practice. Young warned, however, that without internship experience, "the possibilities of reciprocity with other states [is] very poor." Besides, the Arkansas Eclectic State Medical Board might not last much longer. Unless practicing eclectics found some way to help the Cincinnati college, he feared that Arkansas "will fall in line with every other state in the Union and we will have a Composite Board here and naturally the Board then would come under the ruling and rating of the AMA."[57]

Pressure from the AMA was unrelenting. In February 1937, Nellans received a letter from one of the college's outstanding graduates interning at St. Joseph's Hospital in Lancaster, Pennsylvania. The graduate informed Nellans that "the gun at last has reached [him]" as he had just been told that the AMA had removed the hospital from the approved list because of his presence among the interns. The administration of the hospital asked the young man to remain, promising that he would receive a certificate of internship, but requested that he make no mention of the problem to the other interns who were unaware of the change in the hospital's status. The graduate reported to Nellans that he was well liked by the medical staff and was as capable, if not more so, than the other interns. The hospital permitted the graduate to finish his internship but withdrew its offer for him to remain as chief resident the following year. "With the present trouble at hand," he wrote Nellans, "they cannot use me, much to their regret." On a more positive note, he indicated that several prominent physicians had taken an interest in him and felt sure he could become associated with one of them following his residency.[58]

Nellans wrote back to the graduate indicating how sorry he was to receive the news of his difficulties and reported that he had just returned from Chicago "where [he] was again unsuccessful in getting the Council to permit our men to intern in approved hospitals." He urged the graduate to stay and complete his residency and receive the certificate. "I want you to know," Nellans wrote, "that I as Dean have done everything in my power to protect you boys [but] the American Medical Association absolutely refuses to concede a single point."[59] In a final letter, the student informed the dean that he was returning to Cincinnati to open a practice in or around the city. He reported that his residency was near completion at the hospital and, even though "everyone knows by this time, why the hospital went off the AMA approved hospital list, nevertheless they treat me swell and want me to stay in Lancaster."[60]

Some hospitals were abrupt and unyielding in their decisions. One intern received a letter in 1937 from the Passavant Hospital of Pittsburgh noting a recent inspection by the AMA's Council on Medical Education and the warning that graduates of EMC could not be accepted in approved hospitals. Rather than permit the young doctor to finish his residency, the hospital demanded he resign immediately.[61]

Another graduate of the 1938 class wrote a confidential letter to Nellans informing him that, through the efforts of several "friends," he had obtained an appointment in a council-approved (class-A) institution and asked if it was "safe" for him to accept the internship "without fear of being cast out under pressure by the AMA." The appointment, he hoped, would lead to a future research opportunity, but exposure would prevent him from receiving his New Jersey license.[62]

Dean Nellans knew only all too well the difficulties facing his students because they could not intern in council-approved hospitals. Moreover, because so many were Jewish, he was equally aware of the anti-Semitism that prevailed in many parts of the country. In March 1938, Nellans received a letter from C. S. Ordway, director of East Side Hospital in Toledo, asking for information on a particular EMC graduate who, in his application, "dodged the issue of his religion and church affiliation." The letter went on to state that "we have been very reliably informed that he is a Jewish boy and belongs to the college Jewish fraternity." Ordway reminded Nellans that he had spoken to him about "this crowd" several months earlier and asked for an immediate reply, promising to treat the matter confidentially.[63]

In his reply, Nellans indicated that the student had stated on his application form that he was a "white—American" but, since the form did not inquire into religious beliefs, he could only say that the student came "very highly recommended . . . from the departmental heads of the University of Pittsburgh." He informed the director that the student graduated in 1936, passing the Pennsylvania State Medical Board examination with the fourth highest grade of all students taking the examination. He then confirmed that the student, whose father had been born in Russia and was a common laborer, was Jewish. "You know the high percentage of Jewish students at this College," wrote Nellans, "and you also know the difficult time we have to place our men." Fearing that a similar fate might befall other Jewish students, Nellans explained that several EMC students had applied to the East Side Hospital and that some of these applicants were also Jewish. In an effort both to accommodate the hospital and preclude any future graduate from being dismissed from an internship because of his religious affiliation, Nellans asked Ordway to request information on the student's religion before accepting any more graduates of the college.[64]

Another Jewish student described by Nellans as having "consistently ranked at the top of his [junior] class" found it impossible to transfer. Inquiries to Georgetown University School of Medicine and to Ohio State University School of Medicine failed to elicit an acceptance. He was even turned away after offering to repeat his last two years of medical school. Nellans's letters were both apologetic and effusive. "Mr.——, while Jewish has none of the marked racial characteristics, comes from a very fine family with a good cultural background," Nellans wrote to the University Examiner at Ohio State

University School of Medicine. "He is a very mature type of student, serious minded, attends strictly to his own business, is of good moral character, dependable and reliable. . . . Any man who is willing to repeat the last two years of medicine after receiving his degree from this College certainly shows an admirable spirit."[65]

After writing the examiner at the Ohio State University School of Medicine, Nellans also wrote Dean J. H. J. Upham on behalf of the student. He assured the dean that, pursuant to the promise to the Council on Medical Education, EMC had not accepted any more classes and that the school would close June 1939. He therefore asked Upham to consider the student's plight. "While . . . Jewish he is an exceptionally high type man, much more mature than the average senior medical student and is sincerely interested in his work." He would be taking the Ohio board exam in June 1938, following graduation from EMC, but he wanted to intern in an approved institution. Unless he could graduate from an approved school, this opportunity would be denied. There is no evidence in the files that Nellans succeeded in arranging for a transfer.[66]

Final Commencement

The ninety-four-year-old college began its last year of existence in 1938. The seniors were the only remaining class. Nonetheless, the class members stood proud: the student with the highest exam scores on the Ohio medical exam had spent his first two years at EMC and the second highest exam score came from a four-year student at the college.[67]

The eighty-fifth and last commencement exercise for the college was held on Friday evening, June 9, 1939, at Memorial Hall in Cincinnati. After a grand march, invocation, and musical serenade, Dean Nellans presented the graduating class of thirty-six, including one woman, to the faculty and board. He remarked before the assembled audience that monies derived from the sale of school property would be used to establish an eclectic research foundation. According to the dean, the prohibitive costs of operation had ultimately forced the board's decision to suspend classes. He hoped that the research foundation, once formed, would result in the eventual establishment of several endowed chairs in the American materia medica at leading universities.[68] Actually, Nellans's ratiocination was misleading, since the college had never claimed to be an advanced research center; instead, it had historically seen its goal as providing "a thorough medical education at a minimal financial cost." This meant encouraging the college's graduates to become general practitioners.[69]

With the conferring of the degrees by Rev. Louis G. Hoeck, president of the board of trustees, the assembled audience heard an address titled "The Medical Profession of Tomorrow" given by Judge Robert N. Gorman, after which the attendees heard the song "Evening Star" by Richard Wagner, followed by benediction, and recessional. Thus ended the history of the eclectic college, hurried along in its last years by its own graduates who knew only too well that their ultimate legitimacy as physicians depended upon the school's swift passing.[70] At the time of its closure, the college had matriculated more than 14,000, including 440 women, and graduated 4,668.[71]

HELPING THE BOYS

With the graduation of the school's last class, the Council on Medical Education modified its previous ruling by permitting the 1939 class of graduates to intern in council-approved hospitals.[72] Word of this news spread rapidly among prior graduates, who wrote Nellans asking if the approval applied retroactively for the classes of 1935 through 1938. Inasmuch as the curriculum had been the same since the reorganization of the college, they asked why the ruling applied only to the 1939 class.[73] Nellans responded to these inquiries by confirming the ruling and indicating that the council had made its decision based on the fact that the 1939 class was the last class of the college. "I have been very reluctant to make a test to see if the boys from other classes would be accepted in council-approved hospitals until the present class is fully established," he wrote. He saw no reason, however, why graduates of the earlier classes should not apply for a residency based upon this new information. "After all," he observed, "it is up to the individual hospital what they will do with your application."[74]

Equally troublesome to the earlier cohort of graduates was the decision of the U.S. War Department to refuse their applications for appointment in the medical reserve based on the status of the college at the time of their graduation. Nellans wrote to graduates noting that, under normal times, they would not be considered for appointment in the Army Medical Corps. However, "should a national emergency arise, and as a result cause us to be involved in a war, I do not believe any of you fellows would have any difficulty in obtaining a commission."[75]

For the 1935–39 graduates of the college, the surrendering of the school's charter to Secretary of State John E. Sweeney moved agonizingly slow. On February 15, 1942, Roy C. Hunter, president of the Ohio State Medical Board, appeared before the Council on Medical Education to report that EMC had graduated its last class in 1939 and was in the process of divesting itself of all properties. F. H. Arestad, acting secretary for the council, made it clear that any decision to remove the restraints against the more recent graduates of the college would be made only when the council received official notification from Sweeney that the school's charter had been surrendered.[76]

At the annual meeting of the trustees held at the Cincinnati Club on June 19, 1941, Dr. Mortimer Schwartz of Newark, New Jersey, notified the board that the graduates from 1935 to 1939, inclusive, were designated by a delta sign in the directory of the AMA, meaning "not recognized as graduates from an approved medical college." As such, they were not permitted to take postgraduate work for credit and were refused commissions in the armed forces. Schwartz pleaded with the trustees to do everything in their power to correct the situation. Following his appeal, the board read telegrams from six graduates referencing the same situation. However, instead of responding directly to the appeal by officially surrendering the school's charter, the trustees authorized a committee to continue discussions of potential merger with the University of Cincinnati. In effect, the board believed that a solution, short of extinction, still seemed possible.[77]

Hunter, who was questioned almost daily by graduates of the college, found it curious that the trustees were moving so slowly. Writing to Dean Nellans in March 1942, he enclosed a copy of Arestad's letter indicating that the council would remove the inhibitions against the classes "if and when" Sweeney received the school's charter. He implored Nellans to move swiftly, since many of the graduates were anxious to enlist as commissioned officers in the army and navy but could not do so until the school's charter was received by the secretary of state and he, in turn, notified the AMA. Everything would remain in abeyance until the trustees surrendered the charter.[78] On March 9, Hunter again wrote to Nellans complaining that nearly a month had passed since the trustees had stated their intention to return the charter to the secretary of state. "It is my belief that if you folks realized the desperate situation in which these graduates find themselves owing to the fact that this has not been consummated," he reasoned, "someone in authority would see that it is returned at once." He assured the dean that with the inhibitions removed, as promised in his meeting in Chicago on February 15, the graduates would be in a position "to go places." Hunter explained that the school's graduates could then enter the armed forces with commissions and that any restrictions against securing postgraduate work would be removed, including internship opportunities at council-approved hospitals. "I am certainly pleading with you to return this charter at once," Hunter wrote, "for I have every assurance . . . that the AMA meant business and will do exactly as they promised. Please let me hear from you."[79]

On March 19, 1942, H. G. Weiskotten, secretary for the Council on Medical Education and Hospitals, informed Dr. Roy C. Hunter that the college had at last surrendered its charter and that the school was dissolved as of March 17, 1942. Weiskotten responded that the council had removed all "inhibitions which it has made concerning the recent graduates of this medical school." As a result of the council's decision, all EMC graduates from 1935 through 1939 could consider themselves graduates of an approved medical school. By copy of the letter, Hunter informed Nellans of the decision and noted that he had already communicated the decision to "several of the boys who had been drafted and others who had been unable to get commissions." He urged Nellans to give the information as much publicity as would help the graduates.[80]

In response to Hunter's request, Campbell sent a letter to each of the graduates informing them that if they were classified as 1–A for the army, they should contact a Lieutenant Colonel Seeley, executive officer of procurement and assignment service for physicians, and apply for a commission.[81] Those covered by the council's resolution included twenty graduates of the class of 1935, thirty-one from the class of 1936, twenty-three from the class of 1937, thirty-two from the class of 1938, and thirty-six from the last class of 1939.[82]

On June 4, 1942, the Alumnal Association met for the last time. C. R. Campbell reported to the small gathering that the college had finally surrendered its charter to the secretary of the state of Ohio. Since there would be no future graduates of the school, it would "be folly to attempt to carry on meetings." He recommended that the remaining funds of $149 be given to the *National Eclectic Medical*

Association Quarterly to help defray its expenses. He then made a
motion to adjourn. When the motion carried, the secretary jotted the
last words in the minutes of the Association: "Thus closed forever the
Alumnal Association of the Eclectic Medical College. Adieu. C. R.
Campbell."[83]

The trustees eventually sold the college building to a funeral
home and casket manufacturing headquarters and gave the proceeds
from the sale, approximately eight thousand dollars, to Bethesda and
St. Mary's Hospitals. This gesture was made because "the latter two
institutions had been so friendly to the graduates of the Eclectic Medical College."[84]

The Lloyd Library and Museum, the eventual repository of the
school's student records, reported as late as 1964 that the library had
provided bureaus of academic accreditation with information concerning course grades and hours spent in given subjects for graduates
of the college.[85]

RETROSPECT

Intoxicated by the rhetoric of discovery and self-fulfillment that so
pervaded the culture of the early nineteenth century, the first generation of eclectics were as American in their richness and variety as any
group in the tumultuous young democracy. Determined in their protestantism and politically charged for debate, they seldom failed to point
out the conditions within medical orthodoxy that justified their sectarian beliefs. Theirs was a medicine of the head and the heart, an
unequivocal alternative to the perceived failures of allopathy.

As the "mother institute," EMI represented both the strengths
and weaknesses of this distinctive American school of botanics. The
college's early years were a dissonance of temperamental optimism,
alluringly lucid styles, and strong individualism. Rocked by internal
feuds and schisms, the faculty nevertheless promised a worldview based
on the liberality of eclecticism—drawing from any and every source
such medicines and therapeutics found to be useful and unattended by
bad consequences. In doing so, they gave eloquent praise to the French
clinical school with its emphasis on observation and experiment.
Nevertheless, the remark of eclectic Alexander Wilder at the World's
Medical Congress of Eclectic Physicians and Surgeons in 1894 was
more than just jingoistic rhetoric. Eclecticism, he announced to lis-

teners, "is essentially American. It was born on American soil; it was baptized by American blood; it has been championed by Americans during its whole existence. It . . . is American in its conception, American in its practices, and I hope to heaven that it will always be American in its nature."[86] Wilder's comment, simple and straightforward in its expression, captured the unmistakable pride of American eclectics in their system of medicine. Equally important, his comment gave painful witness to the parochial tendencies that eclectics had always displayed—a disposition that gave little more than lip service to eclecticism's broader intellectual origins. Here was a clear foreshadowing of the school's more conservative stance in the emerging age of academic medicine.

When John Milton Scudder took over management of the college in 1862, the ferociousness of the school's early protestantism had been exhausted by too many years of acrimonious feuds and ill-tempered arrogance. Its confidence had been punctuated once too often by frustration and failure. The promise that concentrated medicines would confirm for all time the strength of eclectic practice imploded in the 1850s and early 1860s as school after school closed as a result of lost confidence, financial stress, and the disapproving eye of allopathic medicine. EMI would have faced a similar consequence had not Scudder shown the effectiveness of good management and a more coherent expression of eclectic practice. His theory of specific diagnosis and specific medication, which owed its existence to several earlier homeopathic writers, took form in the copyrighted labels of John Uri Lloyd's specific medicines. Through the careful stewardship of Scudder and the marketing success of Lloyd Brothers, Pharmacists, Inc., EMI and the remaining eclectic schools were able to coalesce around a new eclectic doctrine. As Otto Juettner of Cincinnati observed, "Scudderism [became] a synonym for advanced eclecticism."[87] Juettner's remark was only partly correct; "Scudderism" also became a substitute for synthetic pharmacy and academic medicine.

The faculty and administration carved out a role for their college by giving new meaning to the concepts of family practice, specific medicine, specific disease expression, conservative surgery, and rational medicine. In doing so, however, they turned a half-listening ear to the demands of enlightened pathology and bacteriology, advances in pharmacology, and raised expectations for laboratory medicine. Complicating matters, the management of the college gave clear preference to its own graduates when it came to faculty appointments, a tendency that, over time, caused the college to become increasingly insular in its view of medicine. Alienated by allopathy's continued heavy-handedness and resigned by the lack of political and financial resources to a less important role in the changing landscape of medical education, EMC faced the prospect of justifying its separatist vision to a shrinking number of believers. Refusing to weigh in on the side of stubborn sectarianism and financially unable to modernize fully its curriculum, EMC became not unlike other second-tier medical schools struggling to hold enrollments while searching for a convincing market niche.

Several of the surviving eclectic schools used the confusion created by examining and licensure boards in the states to discredit themselves and their beliefs with scandalous schemes. To the credit of EMC, the trustees and faculty were too honest in their endeavors to participate in these frauds. Instead, the college faced the uncertainties of the future by backfilling its shrinking numbers of believers with marginal students and young Jewish men anxious to enter the profession by steering clear of the admission quotas in Eastern medical schools. Neither of these groups, however different they were in ability, desired to practice as eclectics. Each had been motivated to attend EMC for reasons other than eclectic philosophy and, upon graduation, quickly put down the burdens of eclecticism to join the mainstream of allopathy.

The actions of these graduates, while hardly unreasonable, left the college politically weak and financially stressed. Faced with the shrinking support from graduates who were experiencing knotty impediments to reciprocity, licensure, hospital residencies, staff appointments, and military commissions, the college lost heart. Impatient with the school's inability to obtain an "A" classification, fearful of striking out in a direction that would have placed the college at odds with mainstream medical education, and realizing the bitter truth that the faculty, and not the alumni, had always been the college's greatest source of inner strength, the trustees closed the school. In making this decision, the trustees and faculty ignored their private emotions in recognition of academic medicine's unrelenting demands and the hard realization that, without the support of its alumni, the college could live only at the margin. All that remained of eclecticism were those few alumni who felt betrayed by the decision and who, until their passing, continued to praise the school and its philosophy.

Women Graduates of the Eclectic Medical College, 1853–1939[*]

1853	Caroline Brown	1858	Elizabeth Jones
1854	Mary Malin Bailey		Dora Sabina Wuist
	Margaret Cleis	1859	Mrs. Rebecca Auton
	Mary Eliza Croshaw		Martha Ella Cooper
	Harriett A. Judd		Mary Elvira Morse
	Julia Rumsey		Mrs. M. J. Tanner
	Sarah Smizer		Martha B. Witham
1855	Jane Elizabeth Dolley	1874	Mary A. Ault
	Mary Elizabeth Finney		Anna B. Campbell
	Cecilia P. R. Frease	1878	Joyce F. Hobson
	Martha Ann French		Miranda M. Sargent
	Harriet Hyde	1879	Ida E. Andrews
	Sarah Strickland		Sarah J. Bear
1856	Louisa B. Codding		Sarah A. Booth
	Mary Jane Plews		Jennie M. Lake
1857	Elsie H. Barry		Dale A. Rohn
	Sarah C. Brigham	1881	Havilla C. Hobbs
	Eliza A. Brown		Maggie T. Johnson
	Elizabeth B.Coombs		Ruth E. Newland

[*] This list, found in the archives of the Lloyd Library and Museum, was compiled by F. C. Waite of Western Reserve University and Corinne Miller Simons, Librarian for the library. See *LLM*, Coll. 3, E.M.I. Records, 1845–1942, Matriculation Records, Vol. 6. The original list identified women graduates through 1926. I have completed the list through the final class of 1939. Please note that no new students were enrolled from May 1929 through September 1931 and no classes were graduated during 1930–34 inclusive. Moreover, this list does not include the names of women who matriculated but did not graduate. That number has been estimated at four hundred and forty.

1884   Eva Jane Bennett
        Flora May Betts
        Emma E. Coleman
        Rose V. LaMonte
        Jessie Rose
        Cynthia E. Singleton
        Sarah A. Switzer

1885   Ida E. Andrews
        Mary V. Cosford
        Sarah M. Crosby
        Mary Drake
        Emma Gunkel
        Angie S. Howard
        Maggie M. Kellogg
        Amanda K. Smith
        Mary Williams

1886   Louisa M. Emery
        Lucy Gossett
        Essie E. Haworth
        Emile E. Norcutt
        Mary Potts
        Maud Waterhouse

1887   Mittie F. Bradner
        Carrie Geisel
        Elsa M. Meador

1888   Rozilla Crofford

1889   Lillie M. Myers
        Mary A. Baron
        Nellie Schenk

1890   Hattie M. Fauber
        Blanche A. Guernsey
        Mary A. Lewis
        Eva C. Roloson
        Gussie May Shipman
        M. Maude Sillsby

1891   Laura H. Duncan
        Sarah V. Groff
        Iredale Mary Hobbs
        Henrietta C. Linkenbach
        Elizabeth Miller
        S. Gertrude Norris
        Sarah M. Siewers
        Jennie S. Tarrant

1892   Jessie C. Langford
        Edna T. Matthews
        Agnes Maxwell Tucker

1893   Marinda Lamert Shafer
        Anna Thomas Sheridan
        Flora Williams Smith

1894   Janet D. Quinn
        Maud F. Ruhl

1896   Ella Perkins White

1897   Kate Houseman
        Alexandria E. Walker
        Cora E. Wentz

1898   Lena R. Whitford
        Louise Eastman
        Ivandell Rogers

1899   De Ella Joslin
        Anna Mae Emery
        Mary Beach Morey
        Nannie May Sloan

1901   Florence T. Duvall

1902   Susan R. M. Cooper
        Edythe M. Livingston

1904   E. Florence Stir-Smith

1905   Alta M. Boram
        Etta C. Ieancon

1906	Pina Welbourn
1907	Nellie V. Bradstrat
1913	Georgia B. Sattler Louise F. Richmond
1914	Anna W. Hagemann
1916	Ruth F. Bantum Tressa M. Brandish Margaret N. Dassell Sophie Levinson Maude E. Maltaner

1918	Elizabeth M. Overhulse
1919	Oleen K. Kitzmiller
1920	Ethel M. Johnson
1926	Florence B. MacRae Gayle E. Canter
1927	Atha West Evans
1929	Carmen Thomas Boscoe
1935	Ruth Clark Ferris
1939	Sarah Sydney Schenker

Notes

INTRODUCTION

1. "What Shall Eclectic Colleges Teach?" *Eclectic Medical Journal* 61 (1896): 339.

1. CINCINNATI'S MEDICAL ESTABLISHMENT

1. Charles Cist, *Cincinnati in 1841: Its Early Annals and Future Prospects* (Cincinnati, Printed for the Author, 1841), 14–29.

2. Alvin F. Harlow, *The Serene Cincinnatians* (New York: E. P. Dutton, 1950), 33.

3. Charles Cist, *Sketches and Statistics of Cincinnati in 1851* (Cincinnati: William H. Moore, 1851), 34, 44–45; Harlow, *The Serene Cincinnatians,* 42.

4. Cist, *Sketches and Statistics of Cincinnati in 1851,* 49–51.

5. Ibid., 58–61, 80–83.

6. Henry Ford, *History of Cincinnati, Ohio, with Illustrations and Biographical Sketches* (Cleveland: L. A. Williams, 1881), 293–98.

7. Richard W. Vilter, "Daniel Drake, M.D. (1785–1852): Pioneer Teacher, Author, Medical and Social Entrepreneur of the U.S.A.," *Journal of Medical Biography* 3 (1993): 90–98.

8. From Drake's address "Early Physicians, Scenery, and Society of Cincinnati," quoted in Ford, *History of Cincinnati,* 298–99.

9. William F. Norwood, *Medical Education in the United States before the Civil War* (Philadelphia: Univ. of Pennsylvania Press, 1944), 32–33; George W. Corner, "Apprenticed to Aesculapius: The American Medical Student, 1765–1965," *Proceedings of the American Philosophical Society* 106 (1965): 249–51.

10. J. G. Wilson, "The Influence of Edinburgh on American Medicine in the 18th Century," *Proceedings of the Institute of Medicine of Chicago* 7 (1929): 129–38; Whitfield J. Bell Jr., "Some American Students of 'that shining oracle of physic,' Dr. William Cullen of Edinburgh," *Proceedings of the American Philosophical Society* 94 (1950): 275–81.

11. Norwood, *Medical Education in the United States before the Civil War,* 32; Abraham Flexner, *Medical Education in the United States and Canada: A Report to the Carnegie Foundation on the Advancement of Teaching* (New York: Carnegie Foundation, 1910), 4–5; Nathan S. Davis, *Contributions to the History of Medical Education and Medical Institutions in the United States of America, 1776–1876* (Washington, D.C.: GPO, 1877), 25–26.

12. Martin Kaufman, "American Medical Education," in Ronald Numbers, ed., *The Education of American Physicians* (Berkeley: University of California Press, 1980), 10–11; Joseph F. Kett, *The Formation of the American Medical Profession: The Role of Institutions,*

1750–1860 (New Haven: Yale Univ. Press, 1968), chap. 3; Kenneth M. Ludmerer, *Learning to Heal: The Development of American Medical Education* (New York: Basic Books, 1985), chapter 1; Saul Jarcho, "The Legacy of British Medicine to American Medicine, 1800–1850," *Proceedings of the Royal Society of Medicine* 68 (1975): 25; John M. Dodson, "The Modern University School—Its Purposes and Methods," *Journal of the American Medical Association* 39 (1902): 521.

13. Pierre Louis, *Researches on the Effects of Bloodletting in Some Inflammatory Diseases* (Boston: Hilliard, Gray, 1836); Terence D. Murphy, "Medical Knowledge and Statistical Methods in Early-Nineteenth-Century France," *Medical History* 25 (1981): 301–9; Erwin H. Ackerknecht, *Medicine at the Paris Hospital, 1794–1848* (Baltimore: Johns Hopkins Univ. Press, 1967).

14. Richard H. Shryock, *Medical Licensing in America, 1650–1965* (Baltimore: Johns Hopkins Univ. Press, 1967), 23–28.

15. Donald E. Pitzer, "Standards of Early American Medical Education," *Ohio State Medical Journal* 66 (1970): 366.

16. Quoted in Reginald C. McGrane, *The Cincinnati Doctor's Forum* (Cincinnati: The Academy of Medicine of Cincinnati, 1957), 9–10.

17. Flexner, *Medical Education in the United States and Canada*, 156.

18. Ford, *History of Cincinnati*, 300.

19. Norwood, *Medical Education in the United States before the Civil War*, 306.

20. Ford, *History of Cincinnati*, 301.

21. Norwood, *Medical Education in the United States before the Civil War*, 306.

22. Otto Juettner, *Daniel Drake and His Followers: Historical and Biographical Sketches* (Cincinnati: Harvey, 1909), 126, 129–30.

23. Cist, *Sketches and Statistics of Cincinnati*, 298.

24. Quoted in Ford, *History of Cincinnati*, 301.

25. Cist, *Sketches and Statistics of Cincinnati in 1851*, 113–14.

26. Ford, *History of Cincinnati*, 301.

27. Ibid., 304–5.

28. Juettner, *Daniel Drake and His Followers*, 289–319.

29. Norwood, *Medical Education in the United States before the Civil War*, 322–23; Ford, *History of Cincinnati*, 305.

30. Juettner, *Daniel Drake and His Followers*, 333–35.

31. Thomas Bradford, *The Life and Letters of Dr. Samuel Hahnemann* (Philadelphia: Boericke and Tafel, 1895), 38, 42; Wilhelm Ameke, *History of Homeopathy: Its Origins, Its Conflicts, with an Appendix on the Present State of University Medicine* (London: Gould, 1885), 99; "Hahnemann and Homeopathy," *Medical Gazette* 3 (1869): 109.

32. Samuel Hahnemann, *Oreganon of Homeopathic Medicine* (New York: W. Radde, 1843), 104.

33. Henry H. Hemenway, "Modern Homeopathy and Medical Science," *Journal of the American Medical Association* 22 (1894): 369; Harris L. Coulter, "Homeopathic Influences in 19th Century Allopathic Therapeutics: A Historical and Philosophical Study," *Journal of the American Institute of Homeopathy* 65 (1972): 207–44.

34. Ford, *History of Cincinnati*, 306.

35. Howard A. Kelly, "Some American Medical Botanists," Lloyd Library and Museum, Coll. 3, EMI Records, 1845–1942 (hereafter cited as *LLM*), Eclectic Subject File, box 27, folder 730.

36. Alex Berman, "The Thomsonian Movement and Its Relation to American Pharmacy and Medicine," *Bulletin of the History of Medicine* 25 (1951): 405–28, 519–38; Alex Berman, "A Striving for Scientific Respectability: Some American Botanics and the Nineteenth Century Plant Materia Medica," ibid., 30, (1956): 7–31; Philip D. Jordan, "The

Secret Six: An Inquiry Into the Basic Materia Medica of the Thomsonian System of Botanic Medicine," *Ohio State Archaeological and Historical Quarterly* 52 (1943): 347–55.

37. James M. Ball, "Samuel Thomson (1769–1842) and His Patented System of Medicines," *Annals of Medical History* 7 (1925): 144–53; Frederick C. Waite, "Thomsonianism in Ohio," *Ohio State Archaeological and Historical Quarterly* 49 (1940): 327; Berman, "The Thomsonian Movement and Its Relation to American Pharmacy and Medicine," 417, 420; Philip D. Jordan, "Botanic Medicine in the Western Country," *Ohio State Medical Journal* 40 (1944): 143–46, 240–42; James Breeden, "Thomsonianism in Virginia," *Virginia Magazine of History and Biography* 82 (1974): 150–80.

38. Samuel Thomson, *New Guide to Health; or, Botanic Family Physician, Containing a Complete System of Practice, upon a Plan Entirely New: With a Description of the Vegetables Made Use of, and Directions for Preparing and Administering Them to Cure Disease* (Boston: E. G. House, 1822).

39. Breeden, "Thomsonianism in Virginia," 156–63.

40. John S. Haller, Jr., *Medical Protestants: The Eclectics in American Medicine* (Carbondale: Southern Illinois Univ. Press, 1994), chapter 2; Breeden, "Thomsonianism in Virginia," 165.

41. J. Ben Nichols, "Physio-Medicalism," *Medical Times* 66 (1875): 152–54; Jonathan Forman, "Dr. Alva Curtis in Columbus, The Thomsonian Recorder and Columbus' First Medical School," *Ohio State Archaeological and Historical Quarterly* 51 (1942): 332–40; Juettner, *Daniel Drake and His Followers*, 110.

42. Haller, *Medical Protestants*, 60–63; John W. Shockey, "The History of Physio-Medicalism," *Physio-Medical Record* 9 (1906): 171–81; J. P. Miller, "The Principles of the Physio-Medical System," *Physio-Medical Journal* 14 (1888): 382–86.

43. Haller, *Medical Protestants*, 171–76.

44. "The Farmer and the Eclectic," *Physio-Medical Recorder and Surgical Journal* 24 (1859): 189–91.

45. Harvey W. Felter, "Eclectic Medicine," *Eclectic Medical Gleaner* 1 (1905): 164–65.

46. Alexander Wilder, "Outline History of Eclectic Medicine," *Transactions of the National Eclectic Medical Association* 5 (1877): 40–46.

47. Harvey Wickes Felter, "An Historical Sketch of the Eclectic Medical College," LLM, box 44, folder 1,129; Wooster Beach, *Rise, Progress and Present State of the New York Medical Institution, and Reformed Medical Society* (New York: Mitchell and Davis, 1830), 4–10.

48. Quoted in H. E. Firth, "The Origin of the American Eclectic Practice of Medicine, and Its Early History in the State of New York," *Transactions of the Eclectic Medical Society of New York* 10 (1878): 171. See also Felter, "An Historical Sketch of the Eclectic Medical College."

49. Wooster Beach, *The American Practice Condensed; Or, The Family Physician: Being the Scientific System of Medicine; On Vegetable Principles, Designed for All Classes* (New York: James M'Alister, 1847), 152.

50. Lloyd, "Concerning the American Materia Medica," *Eclectic Medical Journal* 94 (1934): 10–11.

51. J. H. Beal, "Some Aspects of Eclecticism as they Appear to a Majority of Pharmacists," *Eclectic Medical Journal* 91 (1931): 33–41; Alexander Wilder, "Eclecticism in Medicine Defined by Eclectic Writers," *Transactions of the National Eclectic Medical Association* 29 (1900–1901): 95–103.

52. Lloyd, "Concerning the American Materia Medica," 12.

53. Alexander Wilder, *History of Medicine: A Brief Outline of Medical History from the Earliest Historic Period with an Extended Account of the Various Sects of Physicians and New Schools of Medicine in Later Centuries* (Augusta, Maine: Maine Farmer, 1904), 761.

54. "National Confederation of Eclectic Medical Colleges, 1905," *LLM*, Scrapbook, vol. 24, box 43; Harvey W. Felter, "Eclectic Medicine," *Eclectic Medical Gleaner* 1 (1905): 171.

55. *Eclectic Medical College Bulletin* 2 (1911): 8.

56. Morris Fishbein, "The End of Eclecticism," *American Mercury*, July 1926, in *LLM*, Scrapbook, 1927–34, vols. 22–23, box 42.

57. Harvey Wickes Felter, "An Historical Sketch of the Eclectic Medical College," *The Skull—1911* (Cincinnati: EMI Graduating Class, 1911).

58. Jonathan Forman, "The Worthington Medical College," *Ohio State Archaeological and Historical Quarterly* 50 (1941): 377; Harvey W. Felter, "Worthington College, Ohio; Reformed Medical Department," *Eclectic Medical Journal* 64 (1904): 12–13.

59. Harvey W. Felter, *History of the Eclectic Medical Institute, Cincinnati, Ohio, 1845–1902* (Cincinnati: Alumnal Association, 1902), 15; Wooster Beach, *The American Practice of Medicine; Being a Treatise on the Character, Causes, Symptoms, Morbid Appearances, and Treatment of the Diseases of Men, Women, and Children, of All Climates, on Vegetable or Botanical Principles*, 3 vols (New York: Betts and Anstice, 1833), 3:3–4 [advertisement].

60. "The Reformer," *Western Medical Reformer* 1 (1836): 5.

61. Jonathan Forman, "The Worthington School and Thomsonianism," *Bulletin of the History of Medicine* 22 (1947): 772–87; Juettner, *Daniel Drake and His Followers*, 357–58.

62. Announcement, *Western Medical Reformer* 4 (1844): 128.

63. Quoted in Felter, *History of the Eclectic Medical Institute*, 22–23.

64. Felter, *History of the Eclectic Medical Institute*, 24.

65. Between 1853 and 1858, EMI also awarded forty-four honorary degrees for which the recipients were charged between twenty-five and fifty dollars. See Matriculation Records, 1853–1900, *LLM*, Coll. 3, vol. 6; Faculty Meeting, Nov. 1859, *LLM*, Records of Stockholders, Trustees and Faculty, box 1.

66. Felter, *History of the Eclectic Medical Institute*, 27, 38, 45; Juettner, *Daniel Drake and His Followers*, 361; "The New Eclectic Medical College," *LLM*, Eclectic Medical Institute Misc., box 36, folder 1,042. Those schools that enrolled a greater number of students than EMI were the College of Physicians and Surgeons in New York, the University of the City of New York, The University of Pennsylvania, and Jefferson Medical College in Philadelphia. See John S. Billings, *A Century of American Medicine, 1776–1876* (Brinklow, Md.: Old Hickory Bookshop, 1962), 355–59.

2. All the Dean's Men

1. Scudder quoted in "Periscope: Biographical Sketches," *Eclectic Medical Journal* 90 (1930): 184.

2. The ten include Wooster Beach, Joseph Rodes Buchanan, John Wesley Hoyt, John King, Thomas Vaughn Morrow, Robert S. Newton, William Byrd Powell, John Milton Scudder, Johann Bernhard Stallo, and Daniel Vaughn. See Ronald L. Numbers, "The Making of an Eclectic Physician: Joseph M. McElhinney and the Eclectic Medical Institute of Cincinnati," *Bulletin of the History of Medicine* 47 (1973): 158; Joseph Rodes Buchanan, "Reminiscences of Eclecticism," *LLM*, Eclectic Subject Files, box 27, folder 733.

3. Harvey W. Felter, "Eclectic Medicine," *Eclectic Medical Gleaner* 1 (1905): 166.

4. Quoted in Harvey Wickes Felter, *History of the Eclectic Medical Institute, Cincinnati, Ohio, 1845–1902* (Cincinnati: Alumnal Association of the Eclectic Medical Institute, 1902), 88; Ichabod G. Jones, *The American Eclectic Practice of Medicine: To Which are Appended the Posthumous Writings of T. V. Morrow*, 2 vols. (Cincinnati: Moore and Anderson, 1853–54).

5. Alexander Wilder, "Joseph Rodes Buchanan," *LLM*, Eclectic Subject Files, box 27, folder 733.

6. "Clinical Instruction," *Eclectic Medical Journal* 16 (1857): 440; [Advertisement], *Eclectic Medical Journal* 14 (1855): 3. The journal stood for medical freedom, kindlier practice, a more direct system of medication, opposition to the profession being overwhelmed by serums and German synthetics, and resistance to therapeutic systems imposed by allopathic medicine. The last issue of the journal was August 1, 1937.

7. Quoted in Robert S. Newton, "The *Lancet and Observer* vs. The Editors of this Journal," *Cincinnati Eclectic and Edinburgh Medical Journal* 1 (1859): 140–41.

8. Harvey W. Felter, "Eclectic Medicine," *Eclectic Medical Gleaner* 1 (1905): 167. King claimed for eclecticism a large portion of the vegetable materia medica, many of which were already in the official list of the U.S. Pharmacopoeia and had been described previously by Bigelow and Barton. Readers of his work will be struck by the paucity of chemical observations. In truth, the history and properties of the vegetable materia medica received more scientific study by the graduates of the Philadelphia College of Pharmacy than by the experimentations conducted by eclectics. See William Procter, "Review of John King's *The American Dispensatory*," *American Journal of Pharmacy* 31 (1859): 384–91.

9. John Uri Lloyd, *The Eclectic Alkaloids, Resins, Resinoids, Oleo-Resins and Concentrated Principles* (Cincinnati: J. U. and C. G. Lloyd, 1910), 12; Alexander Wilder, *History of Medicine: A Brief Outline of Medical History from the Earliest Historic Period with an Extended Account of the Various Sects of Physicians and New Schools of Medicine in Later Centuries* (Augusta, Maine: Maine Farmer, 1904), 659–60; Alex Berman, "The Eclectic 'Concentrations' and American Pharmacy (1847–1861)," *Pharmacy in History* 22 (1980): 91–103. William Stanley Merrell was a close friend of Morrow and became the institute's official pharmacist, taking up residence in the college, and providing the facilities and equipment for the early work of John King. From 1864 to 1881, he served as president of the Board of Trustees and was known by eclectics as the "Father of American Pharmacy." He should not be confused with H. M. Merrell, with whom John Uri Lloyd was first associated and whose company eventually became Lloyd Brothers Pharmacists, Inc.

10. H. Wohlgemuth, "Fifty Years of Eclecticism," *Eclectic Medical Journal* 56 (1896): 350–51.

11. John King, "Concentrated Medicines Adulterated," *Worcester Journal of Medicine* 10 (1855): 225–27.

12. Ibid.

13. Meeting of Stockholders, Apr. 7, 1856, *LLM*, Records of the Stockholders, Trustees and Faculty, box 1, pp. 161–62.

14. Faculty Meeting, May 26, 1860, *LLM*, Records of the Stockholders, Trustees and Faculty, box 1, p. 207.

15. Faculty Meeting, May 19, 1862, *LLM*, Records of the Stockholders, Trustees and Faculty, box 1, p. 222.

16. John M. Scudder, "A Brief History of Eclectic Medicine," *LLM*, *Bulletin* 26 (1892): 9.

17. John Uri Lloyd, "Professor John M. Scudder, M.D.," *Eclectic Medical Journal* 55 (1895): 3.

18. Ibid.

19. Felter, *History of the Eclectic Medical Institute*, 50.

20. Lloyd, "Professor John M. Scudder, M.D.," 5.

21. John M. Scudder, "On Specific Action of Medicines," *Eclectic Medical Journal* 29 (1869): 393.

22. John M. Scudder, "A Brief History of Eclectic Medicine," *Eclectic Medical Journal* 39 (1879): 305.

23. *Thirty-First Annual Announcement and Catalogue of the Eclectic Medical Institute, Cincinnati, Ohio, 1875–76,* 6; Felter, *History of the Eclectic Medical Institute,* 51.

24. John Uri Lloyd, "Concerning the American Materia Medica," *Eclectic Medical Journal* 94 (1934): 13–14; S. R. Lherman, "The Modern Eclecticism," *Eclectic Medical Journal* 95 (1935): 267; Richard E. Kunzé, "Origin of Medium, or Specific Medication," *Medical Eclectic* 6 (1879): 425–35.

25. John Uri Lloyd, "Specific Medication," *Eclectic Medical Journal* 96 (1936): 25.

26. *Forty-Second Annual Announcement and Catalogue of the Eclectic Medical Institute, Cincinnati, Ohio, 1886–87,* 301.

27. Lloyd, "Concerning the American Materia Medica," 14.

28. Harvey W. Felter, "Eclectic Medicine," *Eclectic Medical Gleaner* 1 (1905): 168–69.

29. Felter, *History of the Eclectic Medical Institute,* 52–53.

30. Lloyd, "Professor John M. Scudder, M.D.," 7–8.

31. "Modern History of the College," *The Skull—1911* (Cincinnati: EMI Graduating Class, 1911): 27.

32. Felter, *History of the Eclectic Medical Institute,* 114.

33. "Modern History of the College," 27.

34. Annual Meeting of Stockholders, Apr. 6, 1903, *LLM,* Records of the Stockholders, Trustees and Faculty, box 1, p. 406.

35. C. L. Olsen, "Reminiscences of College, Feb. 19, 1907," *LLM,* box 35, folder 1,035, p. 7.

36. Felter, *History of the Eclectic Medical Institute,* 65–66.

37. Olsen, "Reminiscences of College," 1.

38. Felter, *History of the Eclectic Medical Institute,* 62.

39. Olsen, "Reminiscences of College," 3–4.

40. Ibid., 8.

41. Ibid., 9.

42. John Uri Lloyd, "Response," *Eclectic Medical Journal* 96 (1936): 199–200.

43. Lloyd's daughter recalled that her father wrote out each of his lectures but delivered them without reading them or, for that matter, using them as notes. The written lectures were torn up after each presentation. Dorothy Lloyd, "A Record Concerning How John Uri Lloyd Lectured," *LLM,* Nellans Papers, box 23, folder 702.

44. Lloyd, "Response," 200.

45. Rolla L. Thomas, "John Uri Lloyd—The Teacher," *Eclectic Medical Journal* 96 (1936): 197.

46. Olsen, "Reminiscences of College," 10.

47. Felix J. Koch, "We Spend the Day with Lloyd," *Eclectic Medical Journal* 96 (1936): 204.

48. Quoted ibid., 206.

49. Michael A. Flannery, "John Uri Lloyd: The Life and Legacy of an Illustrious Heretic," *Queen City Heritage* 50 (1992): 3–14; Michael A. Flannery, "The Apocryphal World of John Uri Lloyd: *Etidorhpa* as a Treatise on the Philosophy of Science," unpublished manuscript, 9. The latest edition of *Etidorhpa* is dated 1994. See also Michael A. Flannery, *John Uri Lloyd: The Great American Eclectic* (Carbondale: Southern Illinois University Press, 1998).

50. William P. Best, "John Uri Lloyd—the Author," *Eclectic Medical Journal* 96 (1936): 191.

51. Caswell Mayo, "John Uri Lloyd as a Pharmacist," *Eclectic Medical Journal* 96 (1936): 193–94.

52. "Triangle of Friendship Broken by Death," *Cincinnati Times-Star* (Apr. 11, 1936).

53. Edward Kremers and George Urdang, *History of Pharmacy; A Guide and a Survey* (Philadelphia: J. B. Lippincott, 1951), 227, 429, 557.

54. Olsen, "Reminiscences of College," 5.

55. Ibid., 6–7.

56. Ibid., 13.

57. Ibid., 14.

58. Ibid., 16.

59. Ibid., 17.

60. Ibid., 18.

61. Ibid., 19.

62. Ibid., 20.

63. Ibid., 21.

64. Ibid., 22.

65. Ibid., 23.

66. Ibid., 23.

67. Annual Meeting of Stockholders, Apr. 2, 1906, *LLM*, Records of the Stockholders, Trustees and Faculty, vol. 1, box 1, p. 412. From approximately 1888 until closing, faculty hires were delegated to an executive committee that, for most of that period, consisted of John Uri Lloyd, John K. Scudder, and Rolla L. Thomas.

68. Annual Meeting of Stockholders, Dec. 19, 1908, *LLM*, Records of the Stockholders, Trustees and Faculty, box 1, p. 417–18.

69. Olsen, "Reminiscences of College," 24.

70. John K. Scudder, Treasurer's Report, May 1, 1912, *LLM*, Minutes of Board of Trustees, vol. 2, box 2.

71. John K. Scudder, Faculty Salaries Report, May 3, 1912, *LLM*, Minutes of the Board of Trustees, vol. 2, box 2.

3. Academics

1. Martin Kaufman, *American Medical Education: The Formative Years, 1765–1910* (Westport, Conn.: Greenwood Press, 1976), 72–149; William F. Norwood, "The Mainstream of American Medical Education, 1765–1965," *Annals of the New York Academy of Sciences* 128 (1965): 486; Leslie B. Arey, "The Origin of the Graded Medical Curriculum," *Journal of Medical Education* 51 (1976): 1010–12.

2. Thomas N. Bonner, *American Doctors and German Universities: A Chapter in International Intellectual Relations, 1870–1914* (Lincoln: Univ. of Nebraska Press, 1963), 23; James H. Means, *The Association of American Physicians: Its First 75 Years* (New York: McGraw Hill, 1961); Robert P. Hudson, "Abraham Flexner in Perspective: American Medical Education 1865–1910," *Bulletin of the History of Medicine* 46 (1972): 554.

3. John M. Dodson, "The Modern University School—Its Purposes and Methods," *Journal of the American Medical Association* 39 (1902): 521, 523–24.

4. Arthur Dean Bevan, "Medical Education and the Hospital," *Journal of the American Medical Association* 61 (1913): 974.

5. Flexner, *Medical Education in the United States and Canada*, 57.

6. Harold S. Wechsler, *The Qualified Student; A History of Selective College Admission in America* (New York: John Wiley and Sons, 1977): 74.

7. Ibid., chapter 3.

8. J. E. Emerson, "The Requirements for Preliminary Education in the Medical Colleges of the United States and Canada," *Journal of the American Medical Association* 14 (1890): 271–72; N. S. Davis, "Requirements for Admission to Medical Schools," *Journal of the American Medical Association* 41 (1903): 409–10.

9. George H. Simmons, "Medical Education and Preliminary Requirements," *Journal of the American Medical Association* 42 (1904): 1208; Abraham Flexner, *Medical Education in the United States and Canada; A Report to the Carnegie Foundation for the Advancement of Teaching* (New York: Carnegie Foundation, 1910): 30–32.

10. Quoted in Simmons, "Medical Education and Preliminary Requirements," 1210.

11. Material quoted from the *New York Regents' Handbook, Eclectic Medical College Bulletin* 5 (1914): 5; "Medical Education in the United States," *Journal of the American Medical Association* 43 (1914): 685.

12. In order of implementation, they were North Dakota, Iowa, Minnesota, Colorado, Connecticut, Kansas, Indiana, Utah, South Dakota, Vermont, Pennsylvania, Kentucky, and California. See "Medical College in the United States," *Journal of the American Medical Association* 61 (1913): 587.

13. Ibid., 684.

14. *Eclectic Medical College Bulletin* 2 (1911): 22–25; Simmons, "Medical Education and Preliminary Requirements," 1208.

15. Flexner, *Medical Education in the United States and Canada*, 32–33.

16. *Fifty-Seventh Annual Announcement and Catalogue of the Eclectic Medical Institute, Cincinnati, Ohio, 1900–1901*, 374.

17. "Medical Colleges of the United States," *Journal of the American Medical Association* 61 (1913): 587.

18. John Uri Lloyd, "The Crisis Is Upon Us," *Eclectic Medical Journal* 78 (1918): 499–504.

19. Letter from John K. Scudder to eclectic doctors, Dec. 8, 1913, *LLM*, Scrapbook, vol. 24, box 43.

20. "Two Years' Pre-Medical Course, 1913," *LLM*, Scrapbook, vol. 24.

21. Letter from John K. Scudder to Indiana eclectics, Jan. 20, 1913, *LLM*, Scrapbook, vol. 24, box 43; *Eclectic Medical College Bulletin* 15 (1924): 2.

22. Letter from John K. Scudder to 236 inquiring students, Feb. 20, 1920, *LLM*, Scrapbook, vol. 24.

23. *Thirty-First Annual Announcement and Catalogue of the Eclectic Medical Institute, Cincinnati, Ohio, 1875–76*, 7.

24. Ibid., 6–7.

25. Ibid., 5.

26. *Forty-Second Annual Announcement and Catalogue of the Eclectic Medical Institute, Cincinnati, Ohio, 1886–87*, 301.

27. Ibid., 299–300.

28. Ibid., 303–304.

29. *Forty-Ninth Annual Announcement and Catalogue of the Eclectic Medical Institute, Cincinnati, Ohio, 1893–94*, 11–12; Felter, *History of the Eclectic Medical Institute*, 61.

30. *Fifty-Seventh Annual Announcement and Catalogue of the Eclectic Medical Institute, Cincinnati, Ohio, 1901–1902*, 273–79. The catalog did not report on the limitations of their students' access to the Cincinnati Hospital and the fact that no EMI faculty held staff positions there.

31. Ibid., 384.

32. "Circular Letter, 1904," *LLM*, Scrapbook, vol. 24.

33. *Sixty-Fourth Annual Announcement and Catalogue of the Eclectic Medical Institute, Cincinnati, Ohio, 1908–1909*, 7, 11.

34. *Eclectic Medical College Bulletin* 2 (1911): 8; "The New Eclectic Medical College," *LLM*, Eclectic Medical Misc., box 36, folder 1,042.

35. *Eclectic Medical College Bulletin* 1 (March, 1911): 13.

36. *Sixty-Fourth Annual Announcement and Catalogue of the Eclectic Medical Institute, Cincinnati, Ohio, 1908–1909,* 14.

37. *Eclectic Medical College Bulletin* 2 (1911): 21.

38. "Modern History of the College," *The Skull—1911* (Cincinnati: EMI Graduating Class, 1911), 30–31.

39. Eclectic Medical College Files, *LLM,* Student Records, box 19.

40. Miscellaneous Outlines and Forms, *LLM,* Form No. 51, box 44.

41. Eclectic Medical College Files, *LLM,* Student Matriculation Records, box 6.

42. Ibid.

43. Letter from Arcangelo Liva, M.D., to Dean Byron H. Nellans, September 7, 1934, *LLM,* Student Files, box 7, series 4.

44. Marcia Graham Synnott, *The Half-Opened Door; Discrimination and Admissions at Harvard, Yale, and Princeton, 1900–1970* (Westport, Connecticut: Greenwood Press, 1979), 44–45.

45. Harold S. Wechsler, *The Qualified Student; A History of Selective College Admission in America* (New York: Wiley, 1977), x.

46. Wechsler, *The Qualified Student,* 157.

47. Hawkes quoted in Synnott, *The Half-Opened Door,* 18.

48. Thomas Bender, *New York Intellect: A History of Intellectual Life in New York City from 1750 to the Beginnings of Our Own Time* (New York: Alfred A. Knopf, 1987), 288–89.

49. Synnott, *The Half-Opened Door,* 18–19.

50. Wechsler, *The Qualified Student,* 169.

51. Jonathan D. Sarna and Nancy H. Klein, *The Jews of Cincinnati* (Cincinnati: Center for the Study of the American Jewish Experience, 1989), 1–19.

52. Leon Sokoloff, "The Rise and Decline of the Jewish Quota in Medical School Admissions," *Bulletin of the New York Academy of Medicine* 68 (1992): 506.

53. "Eclectic Medical College Records, 1845–1942," *LLM,* Student Matriculation Files, box 6.

54. Flexner, *Medical Education in the United States and Canada,* 167–73.

55. John M. Scudder, "Reciprocity," *Eclectic Medical College Bulletin* 14 (1923): 1.

56. Ibid.

57. Ibid., 2.

58. "State Board Statistics for 1912," *Journal of the American Medical Association* 60 (1913): 1638–39.

59. Material taken from New York Regent's "Handbook," *Eclectic Medical College Bulletin* 5 (1914): 4–5.

60. Ibid.

61. Letter from Byron H. Nellans to Maurice E. Scheetz, Aug. 4, 1933; *LLM,* Student Records, box 11.

62. "Eclectic Medical College Records, 1845–1942," *LLM,* Student Matriculation Files, box 6.

63. Letter from W. J. Means to John K. Scudder, February 3, 1916, *LLM,* Student Matriculation Files, box 14.

64. "Eclectic Medical College Files," *LLM,* Student Matriculation Files, box 6.

65. Certification letter from New York Homeopathic Medical College and Flower Hospital, September 11, 1919, *LLM,* Student Matriculation Files, box 15.

66. Student Transcript, *LLM,* Student Matriculation Files, box 13.

67. Letter of recommendation, June 23, 1934, *LLM,* Student Matriculation Files, box 7, series 4.

68. Letter from John N. Simpson to John K. Scudder, Sept. 22, 1924, *LLM*, Student Records, box 18.

69. Letter from Clifton F. McClintic to John K. Scudder, October 15, 1919, *LLM*, Student Files, box 13.

70. *Eclectic Medical College Bulletin* 2 (1911): 25–26.

71. Letter from student to Byron H. Nellans, Jan. 1934, *LLM*, Student Files, box 9.

72. Letter from student to T. D. Adlerman, M.D., Dec. 12, 1934, *LLM*, Student Files, box 9.

73. Letter to C. W. Beaman, October, 1932, *LLM*, Student Files, box 7, series 4.

74. Letter from C. W. Beaman to parent, Nov. 12, 1932, *LLM*, Student Files, box 7, series 4.

75. Letter from Dean Nellans to father, Feb. 8, 1934, *LLM*, Student Files, box 7, series 4.

76. Letter from parent to Dean Byron H. Nellans, Feb. 10, 1934, *LLM*, Student Files, box 7, series 4.

77. Letter from parent to Frank J. Andress, Feb. 10, 1934, *LLM*, Student Files, box 7, series 4.

78. Letter from Frank J. Andress to parent, Feb. 15, 1934, *LLM*, Student Files, box 7, series 4.

79. Letter from parent to Dean Byron H. Nellans, Feb. 19, 1934, *LLM*, Student Files, box 7, series 4.

80. Letter from parent to Dean Byron H. Nellans, Feb. 19, 1934, *LLM*, Student Files, box 7, series 4.

81. Letter from Den Byron H. Nellans to parent, Feb. 22, 1934, *LLM*, Student Files, box 7, series 4.

82. Letter from parent to Dean Byron H. Nellans, Mar. 6, 1934, *LLM*, Student Files, box 7, series 4.

83. Letter from parent to Dean Byron H. Nellans, May 2, 1934, *LLM*, Student Files, box 8.

84. Letter from Dean Byron H. Nellans to parent, May 7, 1934, *LLM*, Student Files, box 8; Student Matriculation Record, *LLM*, Matriculation Records, 1930–39, vol. 9.

85. Letter from parent to Dean Byron H. Nellans, Nov. 1, 1933, *LLM*, Student Files, box 8.

4. Student Life

1. Writers' Program of the Work Projects Administration, Ohio, *Cincinnati: A Guide to the Queen City and Its Neighbors* (Cincinnati: Wiesen-Hart Press, 1943), 69–73.

2. Ibid., 104–107.

3. "Medical Schools in the United States," *Journal of the American Medical Association* 43 (1904): 498.

4. Ronald L. Numbers, "The Making of an Eclectic Physician: Joseph M. McElhinney and the Eclectic Medical Institute of Ohio," *Bulletin of the History of Medicine* 47 (1973): 155–66.

5. William Norwood, *Medical Education in the United States Before the Civil War* (Philadelphia: Univ. of Pennsylvania Press, 1944), 444–46.

6. *Forty-Second Annual Announcement and Catalogue of the Eclectic Medical Institute, Cincinnati, Ohio, 1886–87*, 299.

7. "The Gathering," *The Skull—1913* (Cincinnati: Graduating Class, 1913): 145–46.

8. "New-Year's Night in the Eclectic," *Western Medical Reformer* 7 (1847): 165–68.

9. Joseph Rodes Buchanan, "Reminiscences of Eclecticism," *LLM*, Coll. 3, EMI Records, 1845–1942, Eclectic Subject Files, box 27, folder 733.

10. James H. Cassedy, *Medicine and American Growth, 1800–1860* (Madison: Univ. of Wisconsin Press, 1986), 172, 256; Thomas Neville Bonner, *To the Ends of the Earth; Women's Search for Education in Medicine* (Cambridge: Harvard Univ. Press, 1992), 14; "Female Medical Schools," *Boston Medical and Surgical Journal* 51 (1854–55): 263–64; Richard H. Shryock, "Women in American Medicine," *Journal of the American Medical Women's Association* 5 (1950): 375; Alexander Wilder, *History of Medicine: A Brief Outline of Medical History and Sects of Physicians, from the Earliest Historic Period, with an Extended Account of the New Schools of the Healing Art in the Nineteenth Century, and Especially a History of American Eclectic Practice of Medicine, Never Before Published* (New Sharon, Me.: New England Eclectic Publishing Company, 1901): 570–71; Editor, "The World's Medical Congress of Eclectic Physicians and Surgeons," *Transactions of the National Eclectic Medical Association* 21 (1894): 54.

11. George W. L. Bickley, "Female Medical Education," *Eclectic Medical Journal* 1 (1857): 117–20.

12. Editor, "Female Medical Students," *Eclectic Medical Journal* 1 (1857): 369. Two of the schools where women won degrees in this period were the Woman's Medical College of Pennsylvania and the eclectic Penn Medical University.

13. Regina M. Morantz-Sanchez, *Sympathy and Science: Women Physicians in American Medicine* (New York: Oxford Univ. Press, 1985), 69.

14. Bonner, *To the Ends of the Earth*, 24–29.

15. Martin Kaufman, "The Admission of Women to Nineteenth-Century American Medical Societies," *Bulletin of the History of Medicine* 50 (1976): 251–60; Shryock, "Women in American Medicine," 375–76; William Barlow, "A Case for Medical Co-Education in the 1870s," *Journal of the American Medical Women's Association* 35 (1980): 285–88; Felter, *History of the Eclectic Medical Institute*, 53–55.

16. Newspaper clippings, undated, *LLM*, Scrapbook, vol. 22, pp. 57, 176; vol. 24, n.p.

17. *Sixty-Fourth Annual Announcement and Catalogue of the Eclectic Medical Institute, Cincinnati, Ohio, 1908–1909*, 9.

18. See *LLM*, John Uri Lloyd Papers, box 134, folder 276.

19. "Eclectic Medical Institute," *LLM*, Eclectic Medical Institute Misc., box 36, folder 1,041. EMI offered no student housing and only in the mid-1930s were dormitories made part of the school's master plan—a plan that never materialized. See "Tentative Floor Plans for the First New Building for the Eclectic Medical College as Designed by S. S. and G. H. Godley, Architects, Cincinnati, Ohio," *LLM*, Printed Materials, box 44, folder 1,128.

20. "A Freshman," *The Skull—1913*, 143.

21. C. L. Olsen, "Reminiscences of College, February 19, 1907," *LLM*, Subject Files, box 35, folder 1,035, p. 1.

22. Felter, *History of the Eclectic Medical Institute*, 64.

23. "George A. Baker," *The Skull—1911* (Cincinnati: Graduating Class, 1911): 76.

24. Olsen, "Reminiscences of College," 2.

25. Ibid.

26. Ibid., 3.

27. "The College Calendar," *The Skull—1911*, 93.

28. Saul J. Shapiro, "Graduation Edition," *Eclectic Medical Journal* 95 (1935): 252.

29. *Forty-Ninth Annual Announcement and Catalogue of the Eclectic Medical Institute, Cincinnati, Ohio, 1893–94*, 21.

30. Shapiro, "Graduation Edition," 252.

31. "History of the Class of 1914," *The Skull—1911*, 60.

32. "Freshman Class History," *The Skull—1913*, 79.

33. "History of the Class of 1911," *The Skull—1911*, 50–51.

34. "The Fable of the Freshman who Traveled in High Society, and Believed All He Heard," *The Skull* (1911), 85–86.

35. "Doggone," *The Skull—1913*, 147.

36. "First Offer of Marriage for Student," *LLM*, Coll. 3, EMI Records, 1845–1942, Scrapbooks, 1922, vol 25.

37. Shapiro, "Graduation Edition," 256.

38. "To Horse! To Horse!" *The Skull—1911*, 84.

39. "Organization of the Senior Class," *The Skull—1911*, 38.

40. "Organization of the Junior Class," *The Skull—1911*, 52.

41. "Organization of the Sophomore Class," *The Skull—1911*, 55.

42. Young Men's Christian Association, *Songs of the Eclectic Medical College on the Seventy-first Year of Its Founding* (Cincinnati: YMCA, 1916), 1.

43. Ibid., 2–3.

44. Eclectic Medical College Records, 1845–1936, *LLM*, Photographs, box 40, folder 1,110; "Graduation Edition," *Eclectic Medical Journal* 95 (1935): 263.

45. Shapiro, "Graduation Edition," 261.

46. Ibid., 259.

47. Ibid., 265.

48. "Fraternities," *The Skull—1913*, 85–86.

49. "YMCA," *The Skull—1911*, 74.

50. Football and baseball were not the only pastimes of medical school students. The American College of Medicine and Surgery in Chicago (eclectic) supported a marching band that accompanied its football team. See *The American* [special souvenir issue], June 15, 1904: 9, 23.

51. D. H. Morgan, untitled thesis, 1846, *LLM*, Theses 1848–49, vol. 13, pp. 1–2.

52. Ibid., 5–6.

53. Ibid., 8–9, 11.

54. Charles C. Crandall, "An Original Thesis or Address on the Responsibilities and Duties of a Physician," 1848, *LLM*, Theses 1846-46, vol. 12, pp. 1–11.

55. Nathan L. Van Zandt, "Medical Thesis on the Inferences Drawn From Experiments With Medicine Upon the Impressible Constitution," 1850, *LLM*, Theses 1848–49, vol. 13, pp. 7, 10, 17–18.

56. J. T. Skurdall, "An Original Thesis on the Proper Conduct of a Medical Man," 1851, *LLM*, Student Thesis, box 26, vol. 14.

57. M. H. Siegmund Saches, "An Essay on the True Position of the Medical Eclectic School of America," 1852, *LLM*, Student Theses, box 26, vol. 15, pp. 2–3.

58. Ibid., 5.

59. Ibid., 6–7.

60. "Organization of the Senior Class," 30–51.

61. "Commencement Exercises of the Eclectic Medical Institute, Seventy-Third Session, Tuesday Evening, June 7, 1881," *LLM*, Printed Materials, box 44, folder 1,122.

62. "Eighty-Fourth Annual Commencement Exercises of the Eclectic Medical College, Monday Evening, May 20, 1929," *LLM*, Printed Materials, box 44, folder 1,126.

63. Newspaper clipping prepared by Capitol News Bureau, *Middletown Journal*, June 11, 1928, *LLM*, Scrapbook, 1927-34, box 41, vol. 22.

64. Lyman Watkins, "The Alumni Association," *The Skull—1911*, 16. The association's officers were M. L. Thomas of Harrison, Ohio; N. L. Isgrigg, Moore's Hill, Indiana; B. Gard, Fort Wayne, Indiana; R. W. Hathaway, Chicago, Illinois; and F. J. Locke, Newport, Kentucky.

65. Ibid., 18–19.

66. "Eclectic Medical Institute Files," *LLM*, Alumnal Association, box 24.

67. John K. Scudder, "The Alumnal Association," *The Skull—1913*, 22.

68. Charter of the Eclectic Medical College of Cincinnati, Ohio, signed by John K. Scudder, June 14, 1910, *LLM*, Alumnal Association, box 24.

69. *Sixty-Fourth Annual Announcement and Catalogue of the Eclectic Medical Institute, Cincinnati, Ohio, 1908–1909*, 13.

70. Watkins, "The Alumni Association," 17.

5. Presiding over Change

1. Harvey Wickes Felter, "Rolla L. Thomas, M.S., M.D.," *The Eclectic Medical Gleaner* 1 (1905): 417–18; C. L. Olsen, "Reminiscences of College, February 19, 1907," *LLM*, box 35, folder 1,035, p. 11.

2. John B. Nichols, "Medical Sectarianism," *Journal of the American Medical Association* 60 (1913): 334.

3. Letter from John K. Scudder to eclectic physicians, Aug. 2, 1913, *LLM*, Scrapbook, vol. 24.

4. "Medical Education in the United States," *Journal of the American Medical Association* 63 (1914): 685.

5. "Eclectic Medical Institute Files," *LLM*, Alumnal Association, box 24.

6. Lyman Watkins, "The Alumni Association," *The Skull—1911* (Cincinnati: Graduating Class, 1911), 19.

7. "Eclectic Medical Institute Files," *LLM*, Alumnal Association, box 24.

8. Alumnal Association letter to non-members, Apr. 20, 1916, *LLM*, Scrapbook, vol. 24.

9. Letter from Rolla L. Thomas and J. K. Scudder to 1,620 alumni and graduates, Oct. 20, 1920, *LLM*, Scrapbook, vol 24.

10. "Eclectic Medical Institute Files," *LLM*, Alumnal Association, box 24.

11. Letter from John T. Rouse of Lloyd Brothers to John K. Scudder, May 8, 1923, *LLM*, Minutes of the Board of Trustees, vol. 2.

12. Letter from John K. Scudder to John Uri and N. Ashley Lloyd, May 19, 1923, *LLM*, Minutes of the Board of Trustees, vol. 2.

13. "Hospital Site is Given by Lloyd" (undated newspaper clipping), *LLM*, Scrapbook, box 42, vols. 22–23.

14. Letter from the Alumnal Association to Alumni, Oct. 21, 1924, *LLM*, Scrapbook, box 43, vols. 24–25.

15. Letter from C. W. Beaman to Alumni, Jan. 19, 1925, *LLM*, Scrapbook, box 43, vols. 24–25.

16. "Site for Eclectic Medical College" (Undated newspaper clipping), *LLM*, Scrapbook, box 42, vols. 22–23.

17. Resolution of Board of Trustees meeting, undated, *LLM*, Minutes of Board of Trustees, vol. 2.

18. The minutes of the Board of Trustees discussing this decision are missing from the files of the Lloyd Library and Museum.

19. "Eclectic Medical Institute Files," *LLM*, Alumnal Association, box 24.

20. Letter from W. N. Mundy to fellow alumni, July 20, 1928, *LLM*, Minutes of Alumnal Association, vol. 2.

21. The eclectics were convinced that the automotive manufacturer had a soft spot in his heart for the family physician. According to letters that Henry Ford authored on behalf of the Ford Motor Company to advertise its automobiles, he remarked that country doctors

were "enthusiastic customers" for his automobiles because they were "the first to realize the value of dependable transportation to a widely scattered practice." Copies of his letter advertisements are included in the scrapbooks of the college prepared by John K. Scudder. See *LLM*, Scrapbook, box 42, vols. 22–23.

22. "Shortage of Contry Doctors is Deplored" (undated newspaper clipping), *LLM*, Scrapbook, vol. 25.

23. "Change In Standards Needed to Meet Needs of Rural Health Conditions" (undated newspaper clipping), *LLM*, Scrapbook, vol. 25.

24. "Ohio Physicians on Program at Eclectic Meeting," *Loraine Journal*, (June 19, 1928), in *LLM*, Scrapbook 2, vol. 22.

25. "Specialists Rob Medicine of Bedside Practitioner is Plaint of Eclectics," *Wapakoneta News*, (June 19, 1928), in *LLM*, Scrapbook 2, vol. 22.

26. Nellans quoted in "Says Family Doctor Coming Back Again," *Brownsville Telegraph* (July 1, 1929), in *LLM*, Scrapbook, box 42, vols. 22–23.

27. "Eclectic Medical Institute Records, 1845–1942," *LLM*, Alumnal Association, box 24.

28. Resolution, *LLM*, Minutes of Alumnal Association, box 24, vol. 11.

29. C. S. Amidon, "Report from the Alumnal Association," May 1929, *LLM*, Minutes of Board of Trustees, box 24, vol. 11.

30. Meeting of Board of Trustees, May 1929, *LLM*, Minutes, Board of Trustees, box 2, vol. 2. As a point of reference, N. P. Colwell for the Council on Medical Education and Abraham Flexner for the Carnegie Foundation undertook site visits in 1908, the results of which were published two years later as the so-called Flexner Report. See Abraham Flexner, *Medical Education in the United States and Canada* (New York: Carnegie Foundation, 1910).

31. Special Meeting of Board of Trustees, July 17, 1929, *LLM*, Minutes, Board of Trustees, box 2, vol. 2.

32. Special Meeting of the Executive Committee, Oct. 29, 1929, *LLM*, Minutes, Board of Trustees, box 2, vol. 2.

33. Annual Meeting, Board of Trustees, May 29, 1930, *LLM*, Minutes, Board of Trustees, box 2, vol. 2.

34. Special Meeting of the Board of Trustees, August 12, 1930, *LLM*, Minutes, Board of Trustees, box 2, vol. 2.

35. "Eclectic Medical Institute Files," *LLM*, Alumnal Association, box 24, vol. 11.

36. Special Meeting of the Board of Trustees, Mar. 28, 1931, *LLM*, Minutes, Board of Trustees, box 2, vol. 2.

37. Executive Committee of Board of Trustees, June 22, 1931, *LLM*, Minutes, Board of Trustees, box 2, vol. 2.

38. Letter from Byron H. Nellans to Charles Carpenter, July 12, 1936, *LLM*, Nellans Papers, box 23, folder 699.

39. Special Meeting of Board of Trustees, July 2, 1931, *LLM*, Minutes, Board of Trustees, box 2, vol. 2.

40. Special Meeting of Board of Trustees, Aug. 19, 1931, *LLM*, Minutes, Board of Trustees, box 2, vol. 2.

41. Minutes of the Fifty-Ninth Session of the Eclectic Medical Society of the State of California, July 27–28, 1932, *LLM*, Coll. 18, Eclectic Medical Society of California, vol. 1.

42. Byron H. Nellans, "The Golden Opportunity of Eclecticism" (undated speech, 1930), *LLM*, Nellans Papers, box 34, folder 699.

43. Letter from Byron H. Nellans to R. R. L. Spann, Aug. 29, 1931, *LLM*, Student Files, box 11.

44. Special Meeting of the Executive Committee, Mar. 28, 1932, *LLM*, Minutes, Board of Trustees, box 2, vol. 2.

45. Annual Meeting of Board of Trustees, May 24, 1932, *LLM*, Minutes, Board of Trustees, box 2, vol. 2.

46. Letter from Pearl Montgomery, loan clerk for the student loan fund to student, Sept. 27, 1932, *LLM*, Student Files, box 11.

47. Annual Meeting of the Board of Trustees, Thursday, June 22, 1933, *LLM*, Minutes, Board of Trustees, box 2, vol. 2.

48. Annual Board of Trustees meeting, June 22, 1933, *LLM*, Minutes, Board of Trustees, box 2, vol. 2.

49. Saul J. Shapiro, "Graduation Edition," *Eclectic Medical Journal* 95 (1935): 243.

50. John J. Sutter, "About the Eclectic Medical College," *Facts about the Eclectic Medical College* (Cincinnati: Eclectic Medical College, 1935) 1–2.

51. "The Eclectic Medical College," *LLM*, Accreditation File, box 23, folder 691.

52. Shapiro, "Graduation Edition," 243. Recognizing that more clinical space would be needed, both Nellans and the clinic director explored the possibility of the two institutions erecting a two-hundred bed hospital that the faculty and students could use as their clinical site and obtaining the needed funding from the Reconstruction Finance Corporation. The effort failed. See Annual Meeting of Board of Trustees, June 22, 1933 and June 26, 1934, *LLM*, Minutes, Board of Trustees, box 2, vol. 2.

53. Shapiro, "Graduation Edition," 245.

54. Sutter, "About the Eclectic Medical College," 2.

55. Letter to all matriculants, 1935–36 session, *LLM*, Miscellaneous Outlines and Forms, box 44.

56. Executive Committee Meeting, Sept. 24, 1935, *LLM*, Minutes, Executive Committee, box 2, vol. 3.

57. Ibid.

58. Letter from Marquis E. Daniel to Byron H. Nellans, July 16, 1934, *LLM*, Student Files, box 11.

59. Letter from Byron H. Nellans to parent, Aug. 1, 1934, *LLM*, Student Files, box 11.

60. Letter from Marquis E. Daniel to parent, Aug. 26, 1934, *LLM*, Student Files, box 11.

61. Matriculation Records, *LLM*, Student Files, box 6, vol. 9.

6. Denouement

1. Meeting of Board of Trustees, June 26, 1934, *LLM*, Minutes, Board of Trustees, box 2, vol. 2.

2. Annual Meeting of Board of Trustees, June 26, 1934, *LLM*, Minutes, Board of Trustees, box 2, vol. 2.

3. Letter from student to Byron H. Nellans, July 24, 1935, *LLM*, Student Files, box 6. The note on the letter in Nellans's handwriting indicates that he had a personal interview with the student, but there is no record of an official reply.

4. Letter from student to Byron H. Nellans, June 22, 1934, *LLM*, Student Files, box 8.

5. Executive Committee Meetings, Sept. 24 and Oct. 14, 1935, *LLM*, Minutes, Executive Committee, box 2, vol. 3.

6. Survey of the Eclectic Medical College, Form A, Organization and Administration, *LLM*, Accreditation Files, box 23, folder 686.

7. Dean Eben B. Shewman's job description, *LLM*, Accreditation File, box 33, folder 685.

8. Survey of the Eclectic Medical College, Form A, Organization and Administration, *LLM*, Accreditation Files, box 23, folder 686.

9. Survey of the Eclectic Medical College, Form C, Faculty, *LLM*, Accreditation Files, box 23, folder 686.

10. Ibid.

11. Survey of the Eclectic Medical College, Form A, Organization and Administration, *LLM*, Accreditation Files, box 23, folder 686.

12. Ibid.

13. Survey of the Eclectic Medical College, Form D, Library, *LLM*, Accreditation Files, box 23, folder 687.

14. Survey of the Eclectic Medical College, Form A, Organization and Administration, *LLM*, Accreditation Files, box 23, folder 686.

15. Ibid.

16. Quoted in Nellans, "Dean's Report for January 14, 1936." Rypins received his medical degree from Harvard Medical School and was associate professor of medicine at the Albany Medical College and Hospital. In 1932, he was elected president of the Federation of State Medical Boards of the United States. He was chiefly responsible, along with Dr. Augustus S. Downing, then Assistant Commissioner of Higher Education of the University of the State of New York, for the Webb-Loomis Medical Practice Act in New York, which forbade the use of the title "Doctor" without specific license. The law reportedly forced more than a thousand quacks out of the state in 1927 during the first year of its enactment. Rypins seemed to have been liked by the eclectic college despite his harsh assessment. In appreciation for his efforts in 1938 to place Jewish graduates in residencies in New York hospitals, he was invited to address the thirty-two graduates of EMC at the eighty-eighth annual commencement exercises in Memorial Hall, Elm and Grant Streets. See "Medicine to be Topic at School Exercises," *Cincinnati Inquirer*, (June 2, 1938): p. 16; Byron H. Nellans, "Report of the Dean," Nov. 3, 1937, *LLM*, Minutes, Executive Committee, box 2, vol. 3.

17. Byron H. Nellans, "Dean's Report," Special Meeting of Board of Trustees, Jan. 14, 1936, *LLM*, Minutes, Executive Committee, box 2, vol. 3. Cutter and Dr. H. G. Weiskotten, Dean of Syracuse University College of Medicine, visited EMC as well as eighty-eight other medical schools in the United States during the years 1934–36.

18. Quoted Ibid. The committee's recommendation was reaffirmed at the June 9, 1935 meeting of the Council on Medical Education in Atlantic City.

19. Ibid.

20. Executive Committee Meeting, Oct. 14 and Dec. 30, 1935, *LLM*, Minutes, Executive Committee, box 2, vol. 3.

21. Executive Committee Meeting, Sept. 24, 1935, *LLM*, Minutes, Executive Committee, box 2, vol. 3.

22. Letter to student from S. M. Hankey, Chairman of Intern Committee of Passavant Hospital, Pittsburgh, Pa., May 5, 1937, *LLM*, Student Files, box 15.

23. Quoted in Nellans, "Dean's Report," Jan. 14, 1936.

24. Executive Committee Meeting, Dec. 30, 1935, *LLM*, Minutes, Executive Committee, box 2, vol. 3.

25. Byron H. Nellans, "Dean's Report for a Special Called Meeting of the Board of Trustees of the Eclectic Medical College to be Held at the Cincinnati Club, Tuesday, January 14, 1936," ibid.

26. Byron H. Nellans, "Dean's Report," January 14, 1936.

27. Ibid.

28. Special Meeting of Board of Trustees, Jan. 31, 1936, *LLM*, Minutes, Executive Committee, box 2, vol. 3.

29. Letter from C. R. Campbell to H. M. Platter, Mar. 20, 1936, *LLM*, Accreditation Records, box 23, folder 690.

30. Meeting of the Finance and Executive Committee of the Board of Trustees, May 19, 1936, *LLM*, Minutes, Executive Committee, box 2, vol. 3.

31. Letter from Byron H. Nellans to Charles H. Carpenter, July 22, 1936, *LLM*, Nellans Papers, box 23, folder 699.

32. Letter from Byron H. Nellans to Herbert T. Cox, M.D., July 21, 1936, *LLM*, Nellans Papers, box 23, folder 699.

33. Letter from William P. Best to Byron H. Nellans, Mar. 24, 1936, *LLM*, Nellans Papers, box 23, folder 699.

34. Letter from Theodore Davis Adlerman to Byron H. Nellans, Mar. 24, 1936, *LLM*, Nellans Papers, box 23, folder 699.

35. A. Harry Crum, "Dr. Crum's Tribute," *LLM*, Nellans Papers, box 23, folder 705.

36. Letter from Byron H. Nellans to N. A. Graves, M.D., Mar. 31, 1936, *LLM*, Nellans Papers, box 23, folder 699.

37. Letter from Byron H. Nellans to H. H. J. Upham, Dean, Ohio State University School of Medicine, Dec. 20, 1937, *LLM*, Student Files, box 8. Often, his letters seeking transfers contained offers of "fine bargains" in the remaining equipment of the college.

38. Meeting of Executive Committee of Board of Trustees, Nov. 8, 1937, *LLM*, Minutes, Executive Committee, box 2, vol. 3.

39. Annual Meeting of Board of Trustees, June 22, 1936 and May 21, 1937, *LLM*, Minutes, Executive Committee, box 2, vol. 3.

40. Executive Committee Meeting, Dec. 30, 1935, *LLM*, Minutes, Executive Committee, box 2, vol. 3.

41. Letter from Robert N. Gorman to Honorable John Weld Peck, Jan. 3, 1936, *LLM*, Minutes, Executive Committee, box 2, vol. 3.

42. Byron Nellans, "Report of the Dean," Meeting of the Executive Committee of Board of Trustees, Nov. 3, 1937, *LLM*, Minutes, Executive Committee, box 2, vol. 3.

43. Letter from John T. Lloyd to Louis G. Hoeck, President, Board of Trustees, May 19, 1938, *LLM*, Minutes, Executive Committee, box 2, vol. 3.

44. Annual Meeting of Board of Trustees, May 20, 1938, *LLM*, Minutes, Executive Committee, box 2, vol. 3.

45. Byron H. Nellans, "Dean's Report," Annual Meeting of Board of Trustees, June 5, 1939, *LLM*, Minutes, Executive Committee, box 2, vol. 3.

46. Byron H. Nellans, "Dean's Report," Annual Meeting of Board of Trustees, May 20, 1838, *LLM*, Minutes, Executive Committee, box 2, vol. 3.

47. Ibid.

48. Ibid.

49. Letter from Byron H. Nellans to David McCauley, S.J., Mar.23, 1937, *LLM*, Student Files, box 8.

50. Letter from student to Dean Byron H. Nellans, July 16, 1937, *LLM*, Student Files, box 8.

51. Letter from William A. Pearson to Dean Byron H. Nellans, July 16, 1937, *LLM*, Student Files, box 8.

52. Letter from student to Byron H. Nellans, Aug. 13, 1936, *LLM*, Student Files, box 8.

53. Letter from Byron H. Nellans to student, Sept. 9, 1936, *LLM*, Student Files, box 8.

54. Matriculation Records, 1845–49, *LLM*, Records for 1930–39, vol. 9.

55. Letter from C. H. Young to student, with copy to Dean Byron H. Nellans, Nov. 8, 1937, *LLM*, Student Files, box 7, ser. 4.

56. Ibid.

57. Ibid.

58. Letter from student to Dean Byron H. Nellans, Feb. 19, 1937, *LLM*, Student Files, box 6.

59. Letter from Byron H. Nellans to student, Feb. 23, 1937, *LLM*, Student Files, box 6.

60. Letter from student to Dean Byron H. Nellans, May 13, 1937, *LLM*, Student Files, box 6.

61. Letter from S. M. Hankey, Chairman of the Intern Committee, to student, May 5, 1937, *LLM*, Student Files, box 7, ser. 4.

62. Letter from Student to Dean Byron H. Nellans, Mar. 11, 1939, *LLM*, Student Files, box 11.

63. Letter from Dr. C. S. Ordway to Dean Byron H. Nellans, Mar. 14, 1938, *LLM*, Student Files, box 11.

64. Letter from Dean Byron H. Nellans to C. S. Ordway, Mar. 18, 1938, *LLM*, Student Files, box 11.

65. Letter from Dean Byron H. Nellans to B. H. Stradley, University Examiner, Ohio State University School of Medicine, Dec. 17, 1937, *LLM*, Student Files, box 8.

66. Letter from Dean Byron H. Nellans to J. H. J. Upham, Dean, Ohio State University School of Medicine, Dec. 20, 1937, *LLM*, Student Files, box 8.

67. "Last Year," *LLM*, Scrapbook 2, 1927–1942, vol. 22.

68. "Medical College Sends Forth Last Graduate," *Cincinnati Enquirer*, (June 10, 1939).

69. "The Eclectic Medical College: Historical Statement," *LLM*, College Subject Files, box 35, folder 1,021.

70. "Commencement Exercises of the Ninety-Fourth Annual Session of the Eclectic Medical College," *LLM*, Printed Materials, box 44, folder 1,127; News clipping, "Aged Eclectic College Sings Its Swan Song," *LLM*, Scrapbook, vol. 25.

71. "Cincinnati Medical College Discontinues," *LLM*, Scrapbook 2, 1927–1942, vol. 22.

72. "Annual Meeting of the Board of Trustees of the Eclectic Medical College, June 5, 1939," *LLM*, Minutes, Board of Trustees, box 2, vol. 3.

73. Letter from student to Byron H. Nellans, Apr. 1939, *LLM*, Student Files, box 6.

74. Letter from Dean Byron H. Nellans to student, Apr. 25, 1939, *LLM*, Student Files, box 6.

75. Ibid.

76. Letter from Acting Secretary F. H. Arestad to Roy C. Hunter, President of the Ohio State Medical Board, Feb. 28, 1942, *LLM*, Accreditation Records, box 23, folder 690.

77. "Annual Meeting of the Board of Trustees of the Eclectic Medical College, June 19, 1941," *LLM*, Minutes, Board of Trustees, box 2, vol. 3.

78. Letter from Roy C. Hunter to Byron H. Nellans, Mar. 2, 1942, *LLM*, Accreditation Records, box 23, folder 690.

79. Letter from Roy C. Hunter to Byron H. Nellans, Mar. 9, 1942, *LLM*, Accreditation Records, box 23, folder 690.

80. Copy of letter from H. G. Weiskotten, Secretary, to Dr. Roy C. Hunter, President of the Ohio State Medical Board, Mar. 19, 1942, *LLM*, Accreditation Records, box 23, folder 690.

81. Letter from C. R. Campbell to graduates, Apr. 8, 1942, *LLM*, Accreditation Records, box 23, folder 690.

82. Certification of the list of graduates from 1935 through 1939 by Dean Byron H. Nellans, Apr. 6, 1942, *LLM*, Accreditation Records, box 23, folder 690.

83. "Eclectic Medical Institute Files," *LLM*, Alumnal Association, box 24.

84. "Eclectic College Building is Sold," *Cincinnati Times-Star*, Dec. 1, 1942; "Eclectic Medical Institute Files," *LLM*, Alumnal Association, box 24.

85. Letter from Corinne Miller Simons, Librarian for The Lloyd Library and Museum, to Miss Gladys Lanning, Department of Education, Bureau of Academic Accreditation, Trenton, New Jersey, July 2, 1964, *LLM*, Student Files, box 6.

86. Wilder quoted in "The World's Medical Congress of Eclectic Physicians and Surgeons," *Transactions of the National Eclectic Medical Association* 21 (1894): 54.

87. Otto Juettner, *Daniel Drake and His Followers: Historical and Biographical Sketches* (Cincinnati: Harvey, 1909), 371.

Selected Bibliography

THIS BOOK HAS been researched chiefly from books, pamphlets, journal articles, and the archival files of The Lloyd Library and Museum. To assist the interested reader, I have included a complete listing of books and pamphlets used, as well as of certain general works that afford insight into the period and the subject as a whole, and I have listed all journals cited in the text and notes.

This record of essential materials would not be complete without citing the forty-four boxes of minutes, financial records, matriculation and student records, student files, faculty correspondence, accreditation files, internship records, scrapbooks, photographs of students and faculty, alumni records, and other holdings of the Eclectic Medical College held by The Lloyd Library and Museum (*LLM*) in Cincinnati. A gift of the Eclectic Medical College, the collection represents one of the few complete sets of records left by America's alternative medical colleges. Although some materials are unaccounted for, the collection contains a remarkable amount of information on other eclectic medical colleges, homeopathy, Thomsonism, physio-medicalism, and newspaper clippings on items of medical interest. Those interested in eclecticism will find in the collection a wealth of useful information.

JOURNALS CITED IN TEXT

American
American Eclectic Medical Review
American Journal of Pharmacy
American Journal of Science and Arts
American Medical Times
American Medicine
Amherst Times
Annals of Medical History
Annals of the New York Academy of Sciences

Annual Announcement of the Eclectic Medical Institute
Boston Medical and Surgical Journal
Bulletin of the History of Medicine
Cincinnati Enquirer
Cincinnati Lancet and Observer
Cincinnati Medical Gazette: A Journal of Medical Reform
Cincinnati Medical Gazette and Recorder
Cincinnati Times-Star
Eclectic, and Medical Botanist
Eclectic Medical College Bulletin
Eclectic Medical Journal
Journal of Medical Education
Journal of the American Institute of Homeopathy
Journal of the American Medical Association
Journal of the American Pharmaceutical Association
Journal of the History of Medicine
Loraine Journal
Medical Eclectic
Medical Gazette
Medical History
Medical Reformer
Medical Times
Medical Times and Gazette
Middletown Journal
National Eclectic Medical Association Quarterly
New England Botanic Medical and Surgical Journal
New England Journal of Medicine
New England Medical Eclectic and Guide to Health
New York Medical Journal
New York Regents' Handbook
New York State Journal of Medicine
Ohio State Archaeological and Historical Quarterly
Ohio State Medical Journal
Pharmacy in History
Physio-Medical Record
Physio-Medical Recorder and Surgical Journal
Physio-Medical Journal
Proceedings of the American Philosophical Society
Proceedings of the Institute of Medicine of Chicago
Proceedings of the Royal Society of Medicine
Queen City Heritage
Sanative Medicine

Thomsonian Recorder
Transactions and Studies, College of Physicians of Philadelphia
Transactions of the American Medical Association
Transactions of the Eclectic Medical Society of New York
Transactions of the National Eclectic Medical Association
Transactions of the Ohio State Medical Society
Virginia Magazine of History and Biography
Western Medical Reformer
Worcester Journal of Medicine

BOOKS AND PAMPHLETS

Abrahams, Harold J. *Extinct Medical Schools of Nineteenth Century Philadelphia*. Philadelphia: Univ. of Pennsylvania Press, 1966.

Ackerknecht, Erwin H. *Medicine at the Paris Hospital, 1794–1848*. Baltimore: Johns Hopkins Univ. Press, 1967.

Ameke, Wilhelm. *History of Homeopathy, Its Origin, Its Conflicts, with an Appendix on the Present State of University Medicine*. London: Gould, 1885.

Arber, Agnes. *Herbals, Their Origin and Evolution; A Chapter in the History of Botany, 1470–1670*. Darien: Hafner, 1970.

Aring, Charles D., Albert Barnes Voorheis, and Cory Oysler, eds. *Daniel Drake, M.D. Frontiersman of the Mind*. Cincinnati: Crossroads Books, 1985.

Baker, Samuel L. *Medical Licensing in America: An Early Liberal Reform*. Ph.D. diss. Harvard University, 1977.

Barton, Benjamin Smith. *Collections for an Essay Towards a Materia Medica of the United States*. Philadelphia: Way and Groff, 1798.

———. *Elements of Botany; Or, Outlines of the Natural History of Vegetables*. Philadelphia: Printed for the Author, 1803.

Barton, William P. C. *The Vegetable Materia Medica of the United States; Or, Medica Botany*. 4 vols. Philadelphia: H. C. Carey and I. Lea, 1818–25.

Beach, Wooster. *The American Practice of Medicine; Being a Treatise on the Character, Causes, Symptoms, Morbid Appearance, and Treatment of the Diseases of Men, Women and Children, of All Climates, on Vegetable or Botanical Principles*. 3 vols. New York: Betts and Anstice, 1833.

———. *The American Practice Condensed; Or, The Family Physician: Being the Scientific System of Medicine; On Vegetable Principles, Designed for All Classes*. New York: James M'Alister, 1847.

———. *Beach's Family Physician and Home Guide: For the Treatment of the Diseases of Men, Women and Children on Reform Principles*. Cincinnati: Moore, Wilstach, Keys, 1860.

————. *The Family Physician; Or, the Reformed System of Medicine: On Vegetable or Botanical Principles, Being a Compendium of the American Practice Designed for All Classes*. 5th ed. New York: Printed for the Author, 1844.

————. *Rise, Progress and Present State of the New York Medical Institution, and Reformed Medical Society*. New York: Mitchell and Davis, 1830.

Bell, F. Jeffrey. *Comparative Anatomy and Physiology*. Philadelphia: Lea Brothers, 1885.

Bender, Thomas. *New York Intellect: A History of Intellectual Life in New York City from 1750 to the Beginnings of Our Own Time*. New York: Alfred A. Knopf, 1987.

Benes, Peter. *Medicine and Healing; The Dublin Seminar for New England Folklife, Annual Proceedings 1990*. Boston: Boston Univ. Press, 1992.

Berman, Alex. *The Impact of the Nineteenth Century Botanico-Medical Movement on American Pharmacy and Medicine*. Ph.D. diss. Univ. of Wisconsin, 1954.

————. *A Striving for Scientific Respectability: Some American Botanics and the Nineteenth Century Plant Materia Medica*. Madison, Wisc.: American Institute of the History of Pharmacy, 1956.

Bigelow, Jacob. *American Medical Botany, Being a Collection of the Native Medicinal Plants of the United States*. 3 vols. Boston: Hilliard and Metcaff, 1817–20.

Billings, John S. *A Century of American Medicine, 1776–1876*. Brinklow, Md.: Old Hickory Bookshop, 1962.

Blanton, Wyndham B. *Medicine in Virginia in the Nineteenth Century*. Richmond, Va.: Garrett and Massie, 1933.

Bonner, Thomas Neville. *American Doctors and German Universities: A Chapter in International Intellectual Relations, 1870–1914*. Lincoln: Univ. of Nebraska Press, 1963.

————. *To the Ends of the Earth: Women's Search for Education in Medicine*. Cambridge: Harvard Univ. Press, 1992.

Boorstin, Daniel J. *The Lost World of Thomas Jefferson*. Boston: Beacon Press, 1960.

Boyle, Wade. *Herb Doctors: Pioneers in Nineteenth-Century American Botanical Medicine and a History of the Eclectic Medical Institute of Cincinnati*. East Palestine, Ohio: Buckeye Naturopathic Press, 1988.

Bradford, Thomas Lindsley. *The Life and Letters of Dr. Samuel Hahnemann*. Philadelphia: Boericke and Tafel, 1895.

Brieger, Gert H., ed. *Medical America in the Nineteenth Century*. Baltimore: Johns Hopkins Univ. Press, 1972.

Brown, Geywood, and George Bruitt. *Christians Only: A Study in Prejudice*. New York: Vanguard Press, 1931.

Buchan, William. *Domestic Medicine; Or, The Family Physician; Being an Attempt to Render the Medical Art more Generally Useful, Chiefly Calculated to Recommend a Proper Attention to Regimen and Simple Medicines.* Philadelphia: Joseph Crukshank, 1774.

―――. *Domestic Medicine: Or, A Treatise on the Prevention and Cure of Diseases by Regimen and Simple Medicine.* Edinburgh: Balfour, Auld and Smellie, 1797.

Burrow, James G. *AMA: Voice of American Medicine.* Baltimore: Johns Hopkins Univ. Press, 1963.

Bynum, W. F., and Roy Porter, eds. *Medical Fringe and Medical Orthodoxy, 1750–1850.* London: Croom Helm, 1987.

Cangi, Ellen Corwin. *Principles Before Practice: The Reform of Medical Education in Cincinnati Before and After the Flexner Report, 1870–1930.* Ph.D. diss. University of Cincinnati, 1983.

Carter, J. E. *The Botanic Physician and Family Medical Adviser and Dispensatory.* Madisonville, Tenn.: B. Parker and Company, 1837.

Cassedy, James H. *American Medical and Statistical Thinking, 1800–1860.* Cambridge: Harvard Univ. Press, 1984.

―――. *Medicine and American Growth, 1800–1860.* Madison: Univ. of Wisconsin Press, 1986.

Cayleff, Susan E. *Wash and Be Healed: The Water-Cure Movement and Women's Health.* Philadelphia: Temple Univ. Press, 1987.

Cist, Charles. *Cincinnati in 1841: Its Early Annals and Future Prospects.* Cincinnati: Printed for the Author, 1841.

―――. *Sketches and Statistics of Cincinnati in 1851.* Cincinnati: William H. Moore, 1851.

Cobb, Daniel J. *The Medical Botanist and Expositor of Diseases and Remedies.* Castile, New York: Printed for the Author, 1846.

Coe, Grover. *Concentrated Organic Medicines; Being a Practical Exposition of the Therapeutic Properties and Clinical Employment of the Combined Proximate Medical Constituents of Indigenous and Foreign Plants.* New York: B. Keith, 1858.

Comfort, John W. *The Practice of Medicine on Thomsonian Principles: Adapted as Well to the Use of Families as to That of the Practitioner: Containing a Biographical Sketch of Dr. Thomson: And a Materia Medica, Adapted to the Work.* 6th ed. Philadelphia: Lindsay and Blakiston, 1863.

―――. *Thomsonian Instructor; Or, Practical Information on Thomsonian Medicines.* Philadelphia: Aaron Comfort, 1855.

―――. *Thomsonian Practice of Medicine and Materia Medica.* Philadelphia: Aaron Comfort, 1842.

Cook, William H. *A Compend of the New Materia Medica Together With Additional Descriptions of Some Old Remedies.* Chicago: William H. Cook, 1896.

————. *A Handbook of Family Medicine and Hygiene; Together With Descriptions of Remedies, Numerous Choice Formulas, Dietary for the Sick, Rules for Nursing, etc.* Cincinnati: George P. Houston, 1890.

————. *A Handbook of Practical Medicine: For the Use of Students, Practitioners and Families; Including a Formulary, Medical Ethics and Form of Will.* Cincinnati: William H. Cook, 1859.

————. *Man: His Generative System and Marital Relations.* Cincinnati: William H. Cook, 1890.

————. *The Physio-Medical Dispensatory: A Treatise on Therapeutics, Materia Medica, and Pharmacy, in Accordance With the Principles of Physiological Medication.* Cincinnati: William H. Cook, 1869.

————. *A Treatise on the Principles and Practice of Physio-Medical Surgery; For the Use of Students and Practitioners.* Cincinnati: Moore, Wilstach, Keys, 1857.

Curtis, Alva. *Allopathy and Physio-Medication Contrasted.* Cincinnati: Printed for the Author, 1867.

————. *Discussions Between Several Members of the Regular Medical Faculty and the Thomsonian Botanic Physicians.* Columbus, Ohio: Printed for the Author, 1835.

————. *A Fair Examination and Criticism of All the Medical Systems in Vogue.* 2d ed. Cincinnati: Printed for the Author, 1865.

————. *Lectures on Midwifery and the Forms of Disease Peculiar to Women and Children: Delivered to the Members of the Botanico-Medical College of Ohio.* Columbus: Printed for the Author, 1841.

————. *The Provocation and the Reply; Or, Allopathy Versus Physio-Medicalism in a Review of Prof. M. B. Wright's Remarks at the Dedication of the Cincinnati New Hospital, January 8th, 1869.* Cincinnati: Printed for the Author, 1870.

————. *Synopsis of a Course of Lectures on Medical Science, Delivered to the Students of the Botanico-Medical College of Ohio.* Cincinnati: Edwin Shepard, 1846.

————. *A Synopsis of Lectures on Medical Science; Embracing the Principles of Medicine, or Physiology, Pathology, and Therapeutics, as Discovered in Nature; and the Practice According to Those Principles, as Applied by Art.* 7th ed. New York: A. J. Graham, 1877.

Davis, David J., ed. *History of Medical Practice in Illinois.* Vol. 2: *1850–1900.* Chicago: Illinois State Medical Society, 1955.

Davis, Nathan S. *Contributions to the History of Medical Education and Medical Institutions in the United States of America, 1776–1876.* Washington, D.C.: GPO, 1877.

Derbyshire, Robert C. *Medical Licensure and Discipline in the United States.* Baltimore: Johns Hopkins Univ. Press, 1969.

Donegan, Jane B. *Hydropathic Hyghway to Health: Women and Water-Cure in Antebellum America.* Westport, Conn.: Greenwood Press, 1986.

Drake, Daniel. *Discourse on the History, Character, and Prospects of the West.* 1834. Gainesville, Florida: Scholars' Facsimiles and Reprints, 1955.

Duffy, John. *The Healers: The Rise of the Medical Establishment.* New York: McGraw Hill, 1976.

Dunglison, Robley. *History of Medicine: From the Earliest Ages to the Commencement of the Nineteenth Century.* Philadelphia: Lindsay and Blakistan, 1872.

Dyer, M. Virginia, ed. *American Medical Directory.* 20th ed. Chicago: American Medical Association, 1958.

Eaton, Amos. *Manual of Botany, for North America: Containing Generic and Specific Descriptions of the Indigenous Plants and Common Cultivated Exotics, Growing North of the Gulf of Mexico.* 5th ed. Albany: Websters and Skinners, 1829.

Edwards, J. Jep. *A Compend of Physio-Medical Treatment.* Columbus, Ind.: Edwards Brothers, 1895.

Ellingwood, Finley, ed. *Annual of Eclectic Medicine and Surgery: A Yearly Record of the Observation, Investigation and Experience of the Eclectic Physicians of America, As Reported in Their Papers Presented at the Annual Meetings of the State Societies, with a Condensed Report of the Proceedings of those Societies. Record of 1890.* Chicago: J. M. W. Jones, 1890.

Ellingwood, Finley. *A Systematic Treatise on Materia Medica and Therapeutics With Reference to the Most Direct Action of Drugs.* Chicago: Chicago Medical Press, 1898.

Estes, J. Worth. *Dictionary of Protopharmacology: Therapeutic Practices, 1700–1850.* Canton, Mass.: Science History, 1990.

Felter, Harvey Wickes. *History of the Eclectic Medical Institute, Cincinnati, Ohio, 1845–1902.* Cincinnati: Alumnal Association of the Eclectic Medical Institute, 1902.

Felter, Harvey Wickes, and John Uri Lloyd. *King's American Dispensatory.* Cincinnati: Ohio Valley Company, 1905.

Fincke, B. *On High Potencies and Homoopathics: Clinical Cases and Observations; With an Appendix Containing Hahnemann's Original Views and Rules on the Homoopathic Dose, Chronologically Arranged.* Philadelphia: A. J. Tafel, 1865.

Flannery, Michael A. *John Uri Lloyd: The Great American Eclectic.* Carbondale: Southern Illinois Univ. Press, 1998.

Flexner, Abraham. *Medical Education in the United States and Canada: A Report to the Carnegie Foundation on the Advancement of Teaching.* New York: Carnegie Foundation, 1910.

Foltz, Kent Oscanyan. *Diseases of the Eye, A Hand-book of Ophthalmic Practice for Students and Practitioners, in Which Particular Attention is Given the Treatment of Diseases of the Eye by Eclectic Medication.* Cincinnati: Scudder Brothers, 1900.

Fonerden, William H. *The Institutes of Thomsonianism*. Philadelphia: N. p., 1837.

Ford, Henry. *History of Cincinnati, Ohio: With Illustrations and Biographical Sketches*. Cleveland: L. A. Williams, 1881.

Fuller, Robert C. *Alternative Medicine and American Religious Life*. New York: Oxford Univ. Press, 1989.

Fyfe, John Williams. *Specific Diagnosis and Specific Medication, Together with Abstracts from the Writings of John M. Scudder, M.D., and Other Leading Authors*. Cincinnati: Scudder Brothers, 1909.

Garrison, Fielding H. *Introduction to the History of Medicine*. 4th ed. Philadelphia: W. B. Saunders, 1929.

Gevitz, Norman, ed. *Other Healers: Unorthodox Medicine in America*. Baltimore: Johns Hopkins Univ. Press, 1988.

Goler, Robert I., and Pascal James Imperato, eds. *Early American Medicine: A Symposium*. New York: Fraunces Tavern Museum, 1987.

Goss, Isham Jabez Marshall. *The American Practice of Medicine: Including the Diseases of Women and Children: Based Upon the Pathological Indications of the Remedies Advised*. Philadelphia: S. M. Miller, 1882.

———. *The Practice of Medicine; Or, The Specific Art of Healing*. Chicago: W. T. Keener, 1888.

Gray, Henry. *Anatomy, Descriptive and Surgical*. Philadelphia: Blanchard and Lea, 1859.

Gray, John F. *Early Annals of Homoeopathy in New York*. New York: W. S. Door, 1865.

Haehl, Richard. *Samuel Hahnemann, His Life and Work*. London: Homoeopathic Publishing, 1922.

Hahnemann, Samuel. *The Chronic Diseases: Their Specific Nature and Their Homeopathic Treatment*. New York: William Raddle, 1845.

———. *Materia Medica Pura*. New York: Radde, 1846.

———. *Materia Medica Pura*. Liverpool: Hahnemann, 1880–81.

———. *Organon of Homoeopathic Medicine*. Allentown, Pa.: Academical Bookstore, 1836.

Hall, Marshall. *Observations on Blood-Letting Founded Upon Researches on the Morbid and Curative Effects of Loss of Blood*. London: Sherwood, 1836.

Haller, Jr., John S. *American Medicine in Transition, 1840–1910*. Urbana: Univ. of Illinois Press, 1981.

———. *Kindly Medicine: Physio-Medicalism in America, 1836–1911*. Kent, Ohio: Kent State Univ. Press, 1997.

———. *Medical Protestants: The Eclectics in American Medicine, 1825–1939*. Carbondale: Southern Illinois Univ. Press, 1994.

Hardwicke, Herbert Junius. *Medical Education and Practice in All Parts of the World*. Philadelphia: Presley Blakiston, 1880.

Harlow, Alvin F. *The Serene Cincinnatians*. New York: E. P. Dutton, 1950.

Harvey, A. McGehee. *Adventures in Medical Research: A Century of Discovery at Johns Hopkins*. Baltimore: Johns Hopkins Univ. Press, 1976.

————. *Science at the Bedside: Clinical Research in American Medicine, 1905–1945*. Baltimore: Johns Hopkins Univ. Press, 1981.

Hein, Wolfgang-Gagen, ed. *Botanical Drugs of the Americas in the Old and New Worlds*. Stuttgart: Wissenschaftliche Verlagsgesellschaft MBH, 1984.

Henry, Samuel. *A New and Complete Family Herbal*. New York: Printed for the Author, 1814.

Hoener, Frederick G. *The New Physiologic Medication*. 2d ed. Baltimore: Printed for the Author, 1900.

House, Eleazer G. *The Botanic Family Friend: Being a Complete Guide to the New System of Thomsonian Medical Practice*. Boston: Printed for the Author, 1844.

Howard, Horton. *An Improved System of Botanic Medicine Founded Upon Correct Physiological Principles; Comprising a Complete Treatise on the Practice of Medicine*. Cincinnati: Kost, Bigger and Hart, 1832.

Howe, Andrew Jackson. *The Art and Science of Surgery*. Cincinnati: Wilstach, Baldwin, 1876.

————. *Manual of Eye Surgery*. Cincinnati: Wilstach, Baldwin, 1874.

————. *Miscellaneous Papers by Andrew Jackson Howe Selected and Arranged by his Wife, Georgiana L. Howe*. Cincinnati: Robert Clarke, 1894.

————. *Operative Gynacology*. Cincinnati: Robert Clarke, 1890.

————. *A Practical and Systematic Treatise on Fractures and Dislocations*. Cincinnati: J. M. Scudder, 1891.

Illinois State Board of Health. *Report on Medical Education and the Regulation of the Practice of Medicine in the United States and Canada*. Springfield, Ill.: State Board of Health, 1883.

Jahr, Gottlieb Heinrich. *Hull's Jahr; A New Manual of Homeopathic Practice*. New York: Radde, 1862.

Jeancon, John A. *Diseases of the Sexual Organs, Male and Female. Anatomy, Normal and Morbid; Pathology, Physical Diagnosis and Treatment of the Diseases of Those Organs*. Cincinnati: Pathological Publishing, 1894.

————. *Explanatory Text to the Atlas of Human Anatomy*. Cincinnati: Wilde, 1880.

————. *Pathological Anatomy, Pathology and Diagnosis: A Series of Clinical Reports Comprising the Principal Diseases of the Human Body*. Cincinnati: Progress Publishing, 1882.

Jones, Ichabod Gibson. *The American Eclectic Practice of Medicine: To Which Are Appended the Posthumous Writings of T. V. Morrow*. Cincinnati: Moore, Anderson, 1853–54.

Jones, Lorenzo E. and John M. Scudder. *The American Eclectic Materia Medica and Therapeutics*. Cincinnati: Moore, Wilstach, Keys, 1858–59.

Juettner, Otto. *Daniel Drake and His Followers: Historical and Biographical Sketches*. Cincinnati: Harvey, 1909.

Kaufman, Martin. *American Medical Education: The Formative Years, 1765–1910*. Westport, Conn.: Greenwood Press, 1976.

———. *Homeopathy in America: The Rise and Fall of a Medical Heresy*. Baltimore: Johns Hopkins Univ. Press, 1971.

Kaufman, Martin, Stewart Gailishoff, and Todd L. Savitt, eds. *Dictionary of American Medical Biography*. 2 vols. Westport, Conn.: Greenwood Press, 1984.

Keith, Melville C. *Keith's Domestic Practice and Botanic Hand Book*. Bellville, Ohio: Printed for the Author, 1901.

Kett, F. Joseph. *The Formation of the American Medical Profession*. New Haven: Yale University Press, 1968.

King, John. *The American Eclectic Dispensatory*. Cincinnati: Moore, Wilstach, Keys, 1870.

———. *King's American Dispensatory*. Cincinnati: The Ohio Valley Company, 1898–1900.

Kirkes, William Senhouse. *Handbook of Physiology*. 4th ed. London: Walton and Maberly, 1860.

Kost, John. *Domestic Medicine: A Treatise on the Practice of Medicine Adapted to the Reformed System, Comprising a Materia Medica*. Cincinnati: Burnard, 1851.

———. *Elements of the Materia Medica and Therapeutics: Adapted to the New Physiological System of Practice*. Cincinnati: Kost and Pool, 1849.

———. *The Practice of Medicine According to the Plan Most Approved by the Reformed or Botanic Colleges of the United States, Embracing a Treatise on Materia Medica and Pharmacy, Designed Principally for Families*. Mt. Vernon, Ohio: N. p., 1847.

Lloyd, John Uri. *The Chemistry of Medicines, Practical: A Text and Reference Book for the Use of Students, Physicians, and Pharmacists, Embodying the Principles of Chemical Philosophy and their Application to those Chemicals*. Cincinnati: Robert Clarke, 1881.

———. *Drugs and Medicines of North America: A Publication Devoted to the Historical and Scientific Discussion of Botany, Pharmacy, Chemistry and Therapeutics of the Medical Plants of North America*. Cincinnati: J. U. Lloyd and C. G. Lloyd, 1884–87.

———. *The Eclectic Alkaloids, Resins, Resinoids, Oleo-Resins and Concentrated Principles*. Cincinnati: J. U. and C. G. Lloyd, 1910.

———. *History of the Vegetable Drugs of the Pharmacopoeia of the United States*. Cincinnati: J. U. and C. G. Lloyd, 1911.

———. *Origin and History of All the Pharmacopeial Vegetable Drugs, Chemicals and Preparations*. Cincinnati: Caxton Press, 1921.

Lloyd, John Uri, and C. G. Lloyd. *Drugs and Medicines of North America: A Publication Devoted to the Historical and Scientific Discussion of Botany, Pharmacy, Chemistry and Therapeutics of the Medical Plants of North America.* Cincinnati: J. U. Lloyd and C. G. Lloyd, 1884–87.

Lopate, Carol. *Women in Medicine*. Baltimore: Johns Hopkins Univ. Press, 1968.

Louis, Pierre. *Researches on the Effects of Bloodletting in Some Inflammatory Diseases*. Boston: Hilliard, Gray, 1836.

Ludmerer, Kenneth M. *Learning to Heal: The Development of American Medical Education*. New York: Basic Books, 1985.

Lyle, T. J. *Physio-Medical Therapeutics, Materia Medica, and Pharmacy*. Salem, Ohio: J. M. Lyle and Brothers, 1897.

Mattson, Morris. *The American Vegetable Practice: Or, A New and Improved Guide to Health, Designed for the Use of Families*. 2 vols. Boston: Daniel L. Hale, 1841.

Means, James H. *The Association of American Physicians: Its First 75 Years*. New York: McGraw Hill, 1961.

Morantz-Sanchez, Regina. *Sympathy and Science: Women Physicians in American Medicine*. New York: Oxford Univ. Press, 1985.

Murphy, Lamar R. *Enter the Physician: The Transformation of Domestic Medicine, 1760–1860*. Tuscaloosa: Univ. of Alabama Press, 1991.

Newton, Robert Safford. *An Eclectic Treatise on the Practice of Medicine: Embracing the Pathology of Inflammation and Fever, with Its Classification and Treatment*. Cincinnati: N. p., 1861.

Niederkorn, Joseph Stephen. *A Handy Reference Book: Giving Briefly the Specific Indication for Remedies, Paying Particular Attention to Each Organ of the Body Distinctively*. Cincinnati, Ohio: Printed for the Author, 1905.

Nissenbaum, Stephen. *Sex, Diet, and Debility in Jacksonian America: Sylvester Graham and Health Reform*. Westport, Conn.: Greenwood Press, 1980.

Norwood, William F. *Medical Education in the United States Before the Civil War*. Philadelphia: Univ. of Pennsylvania Press, 1944.

Numbers, Ronald, ed. *The Education of American Physicians*. Berkeley: Univ. of California Press, 1980.

Oesterreicher, Johann Heinrich. *Atlas of Human Anatomy, Containing 197 Large Plates Taken from the Original Designs from Nature*. Cincinnati: A. E. Wilde, 1879–85.

———. *Explanatory Text to the Atlas of Human Anatomy*. Cincinnati: A. E. Wilde, 1885.

Paine, William. *An Epitome of the American Eclectic Practice of Medicine: Embracing Pathology, Symptomatology, Diagnosis, Prognosis and Treatment*. Philadelphia: H. Cowperthwaite, 1857.

———. *An Epitome of the American Eclectic Practice of Medicine, Surgery, Obstetrics, Diseases of Women and Children, Materia Medica and Pharmacy, with Glossary*. Philadelphia: J. Gladding, 1859.

Pickard, Madge E., and R. Carlyle Buley. *The Midwest Pioneer: His Ills, Cures, and Doctors*. New York: Henry Schuman, 1946.

Polk's Medical Register and Directory of North America. Detroit: R. L. Polk, 1886–1906.

Powell, William Byrd. *The Eclectic Practice of Medicine: Diseases of Children*. Cincinnati: Rickey, Mallory, 1858.

Poynter, F. N. L. *Medicine and Science in the 1860s: Proceedings of the 6th British Congress on the History of Medicine*. London: Welcome Institute for the History of Medicine, 1968.

Rafinesque, Constantine S. *Medical Flora: Or, Manual of the Medical Botany of the United States of North America*. 2 vols. Philadelphia: Atkinson and Alexander, 1828–30.

Reed, Louis S. *The Healing Cults; A Study of Sectarian Medical Practice: Its Extent, Causes, and Control*. Chicago: Univ. of Chicago Press, 1932.

Risse, Guenter B., Ronald L. Numbers, and Judith W. Leavitt, eds. *Medicine Without Doctors: Home Health Care in American History*. New York: Science History, 1977.

Rothstein, William G. *American Physicians in the Nineteenth Century: From Sects to Science*. Baltimore: Johns Hopkins Univ. Press, 1972.

Sarna, Jonathan D., and Nancy H. Klein. *The Jews of Cincinnati*. Cincinnati: Center for the Study of the American Jewish Experience, 1989.

Scudder, John M. *The Eclectic Practice of Medicine*. Cincinnati: Moore, Wilstach, Keys, 1864.

———. *The Eclectic Practice of Medicine*. Cincinnati: Medical Publishing, 1870.

———. *On the Reproductive Organs and the Venereal*. Cincinnati: Wilstach, Baldwin, 1874.

———. *On the Use of Medicated Inhalations, in the Treatment of Diseases of the Respiratory Organs*. Cincinnati: Moore, Wilstach and Baldwin, 1867.

———. *The Principles of Medicine*. Cincinnati: Moore, Wilstach and Baldwin, 1867.

———. *Specific Diagnosis: A Study of Disease, With Special Reference to the Administration of Remedies*. Cincinnati: Wilstach, Baldwin, 1883.

———. *Specific Medication and Specific Medicines: Revised, with an Appendix Containing the Articles Published on the Subject Since the First Edition; and a*

Report of Cases Illustrating Specific Medication. Cincinnati: Wilstach, Baldwin, 1873.

———. *Specific Medication and Specific Medicines*. Cincinnati: Wilstach, Baldwin, 1884.

Shafer, Henry B. *The American Medical Profession: 1783–1850*. New York: Columbia Univ. Press, 1936.

Shryock, Richard H. *The Development of Modern Medicine: An Interpretation of the Social and Scientific Factors Involved*. Philadelphia: Univ. of Pennsylvania Press, 1936.

———. *Medical Licensing in America, 1650–1965*. Baltimore: Johns Hopkins Univ. Press, 1967.

The Skull—1911. Cincinnati: Graduating Class of the Eclectic Medical Institute, 1911.

The Skull—1913. Cincinnati: Graduating Class of the Eclectic Medical Institute, 1913.

Smith, Elias. *The American Physician and Family Assistant*. Boston: E. Bellamy, 1826.

———. *The Medical Pocket-Book: Family Physician and Sick Man's Guide to Health*. Boston: Henry Bowen, 1822.

Smith, Elisha. *The Botanic Physician: Being a Compendium of the Practice of Physic, upon Botanical Principles*. New York: Murphy and Bingham, 1830.

Sonnedecker, Glenn. *Kremers and Urdang's History of Pharmacy*. 3d ed. Philadelphia: J. B. Lippincott, 1963.

Starr, Paul E. *The Social Transformation of American Medicine: The Rise of a Sovereign Profession and the Making of a Vast Industry*. New York: Basic Books, 1982.

Steele, Joel Dorman. *Fourteen Weeks in Physics*. New York: A. S. Barnes, 1878.

Sutter, John J. *Facts About the Eclectic Medical College*. Cincinnati: Eclectic Medical College, 1935.

Synnott, Marcia Graham. *The Half-Opened Door: Discrimination and Admissions at Harvard, Yale, and Princeton, 1900–1970*. Westport, Conn.: Greenwood Press, 1979.

Tenney, Sanborn. *Natural History: A Manual of Zoology for Schools, Colleges, and the General Reader*. New York: Charles Scribner, 1865.

Thomson, John. *A Historical Sketch of the Thomsonian System of the Practice of Medicine on Botanical Principles*. Albany: B. D. Packard, 1830.

———. *A Vindication of the Thomsonian System of Practice of Medicine on Botanical Principles*. Albany: Webster and Wood, 1825.

Thomson, Samuel. *New Guide to Health: Or, Botanic Family Physician, Containing a Complete System of Practice, Upon a Plan Entirely New: With a*

Description of the Vegetables Made Use of, and Directions for Preparing and Administering Them to Cure Disease. Boston: E. G. House, 1822.

———. *The Thomsonian Materia Medica or Botanic Family Physician: Comprising a Philosophical Theory, the Natural Organization and Assumed Principles of Animal and Vegetable Life: To Which are Added the Description of Plants.* 12th ed. Albany: J. Munsell, 1841.

Thurston, Joseph M. *The Philosophy of Physiomedicalism. Its Theorem, Corollary, and Laws of Application for the Cure of Disease.* Richmond, Indiana: Nicholson, 1900.

———. *The Principia of Medicine: A Universal Working Hypothesis for a Medical Science.* Richmond, Ind.: J. M. Thurston, 1896.

Veysey, Lawrence R. *The Emergence of the American University.* Chicago: Univ. of Chicago Press, 1965.

Victor, John. *A History of the Council on Medical Education and Hospitals of the AMA, 1904–1959.* Chicago: AMA, 1959.

Walsh, Mary Roth. *Doctors Wanted: No Women Need Apply; Sexual Barriers in the Medical Profession, 1835–1975.* New Haven: Yale Univ. Press, 1977.

Warner, John H. *The Therapeutic Perspective; Medical Practice, Knowledge, and Identity in America, 1820–1880.* Cambridge: Harvard Univ. Press, 1986.

Webster, Herbert Tracy. *Dynamical Therapeutics.* Oakland, Calif.: Printed for the Author, 1893.

———. *New Eclectic Medical Practice; Designed for Students and Practitioners.* Oakland, Calif.: Webster Medical, 1899.

———. *The Principles of Medicine as Applied to Dynamical Therapeutics.* Oakland, Calif.: Printed for the Author, 1891.

Wechsler, Harold S. *The Qualified Student; A History of Selective College Admission in America.* New York: John Wiley and Sons, 1977.

Weiss, Harry B., and Howard R. Kemble. *The Great American Water-Cure Craze: A History of Hydropathy in the United States.* Trenton, N.J.: Past Times Press, 1967.

Wilder, Alexander. *A History of Medicine: A Brief Outline of Medical History from the Earliest Historic Period with an Extended Account of the Various Sects of Physicians and New Schools of Medicine in Later Centuries.* Augusta, Maine: Maine Farmer, 1904.

Wilson, Cloyce. *Useful Prescriptions.* Cincinnati: Lloyd Brothers, Pharmacists, 1935.

Wilson, W. *Practice of Medicine on Thomsonian Principles.* Memphis, Tenn.: W. Wilson, 1855.

Wood, George B., and Franklin Bache. *The Dispensatory of the United States of America.* Philadelphia: Lippincott, 1866.

Worthy, A. N. *A Treatise on the Botanic Theory and Practice of Medicine*. Forsythe, Ga.: C. R. Hareleiter, 1842.

Writers' Program of the Work Projects Administration, Ohio. *Cincinnati: A Guide to the Queen City and Its Neighbors*. Cincinnati: Wiesen-Hart Press, 1943.

Young Men's Christian Association. *Songs of the Eclectic Medical College on the Seventy-first Year of Its Founding*. Cincinnati: YMCA, 1916.

Index